M000287841

VITAMINS
& SUPPLEMENTS
From
A *to* Z
Boost Your Immunity
& Never Get Sick!

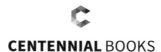
CENTENNIAL BOOKS

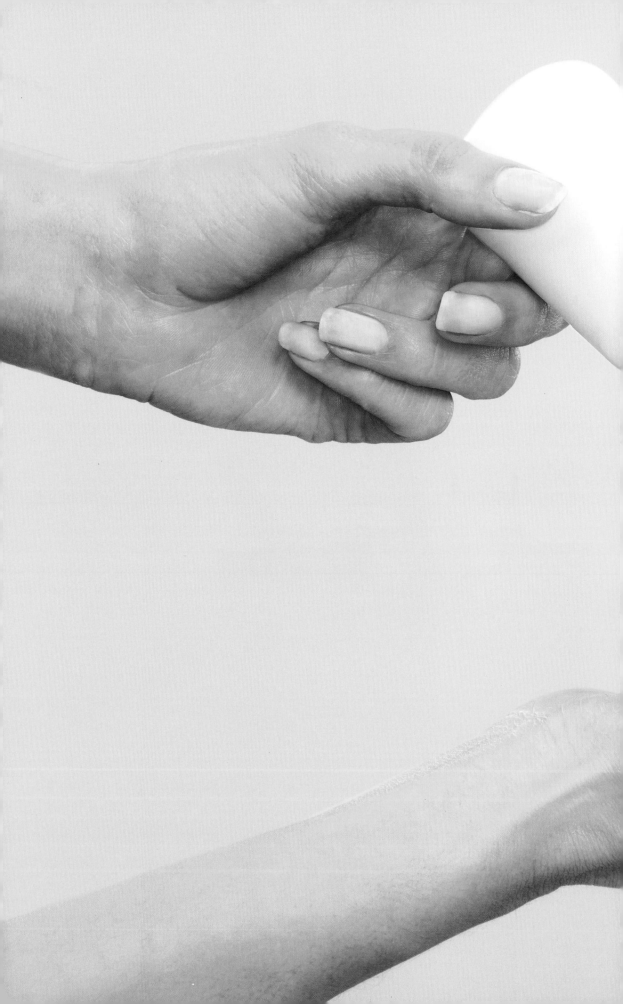

VITAMINS
& SUPPLEMENTS

From

A *to* Z

Boost Your Immunity
& Never Get Sick!

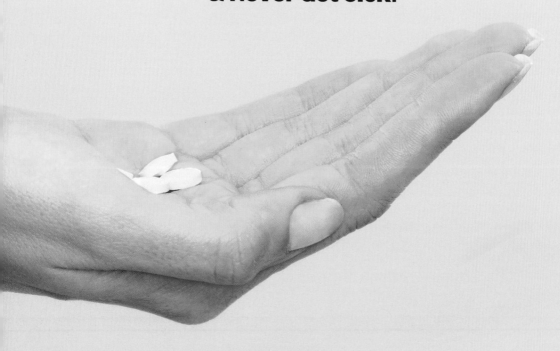

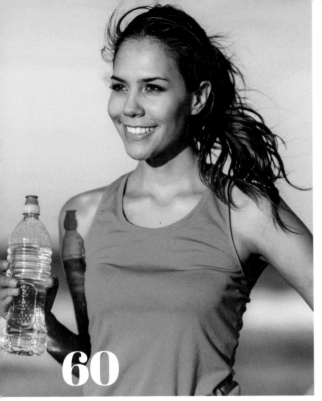

60

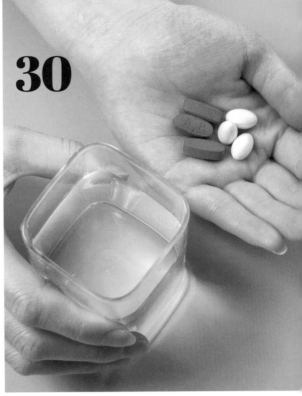

30

Contents

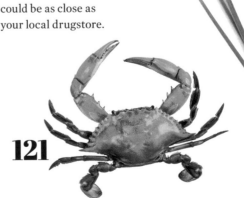

108

6 Introduction
Learn how to navigate the
wild world of supplements.

Chapter 1
**WHAT NUTRIENTS
CAN DO FOR YOU**
**10 The Body's
Building Blocks**
How vitamins and minerals
keep you strong and healthy.

18 Stick to Food
Some nutrients are just
better when you eat them.
Here's a list of what matters.

**24 Who Really
Needs Supplements?**
If you happen to be
pregnant, are a picky eater
or are over a certain age, you
likely need a supplement.

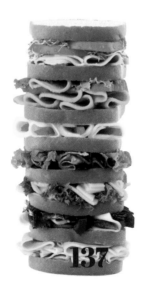

137

**30 The Most
Common Deficiencies**
Watch out for these
symptoms—they could
indicate you're dangerously
low on key nutrients.

**40 Know Your
Nutrient Limits**
Too much of a good
thing can actually
become dangerous,
so be sure to stay safe
with your choices.

Chapter 2
**THE POWER OF
SUPPLEMENTS**
48 Stay Young
The fountain of youth
could be as close as
your local drugstore.

121

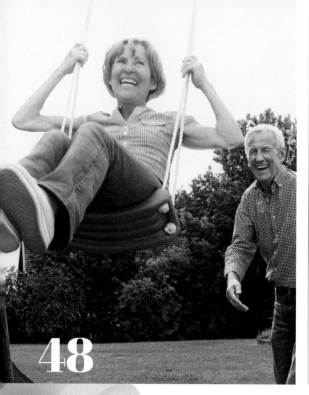

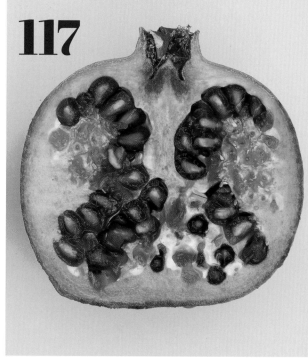

117

48

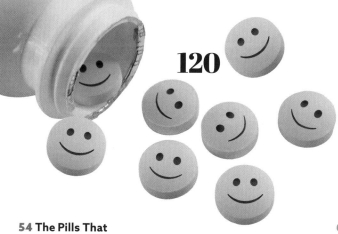

120

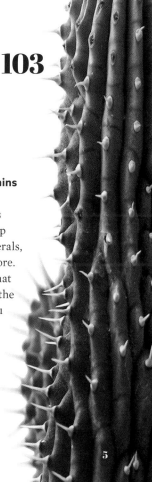

103

**54 The Pills That
Help You Shed Pounds**
Everyone knows how tough
it is to lose weight. Here's
the extra help you need to
make the loss stick this time.

**60 Fight Fatigue
& Get Your Energy Back**
Dragging and lagging
through your day is no way
to live. Time to get your
oomph going again.

66 Libido Boosters
How to add some pep
back in your bedroom life
without pharmaceuticals.

**68 Smart Ways
to Stay Sharp**
A stronger memory,
a mind that responds
well even under pressure
and protection against
dementia, all within reach.

**Chapter 3
THE ESSENTIAL
A TO Z GUIDE
76 99 Important Vitamins
& Supplements**
From acai to zinc, here's
an encyclopedic roundup
of all the vitamins, minerals,
herbs, probiotics and more.
Learn what they are, what
they can do for you and the
amounts experts say you
need to stay healthy.

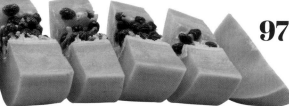

97

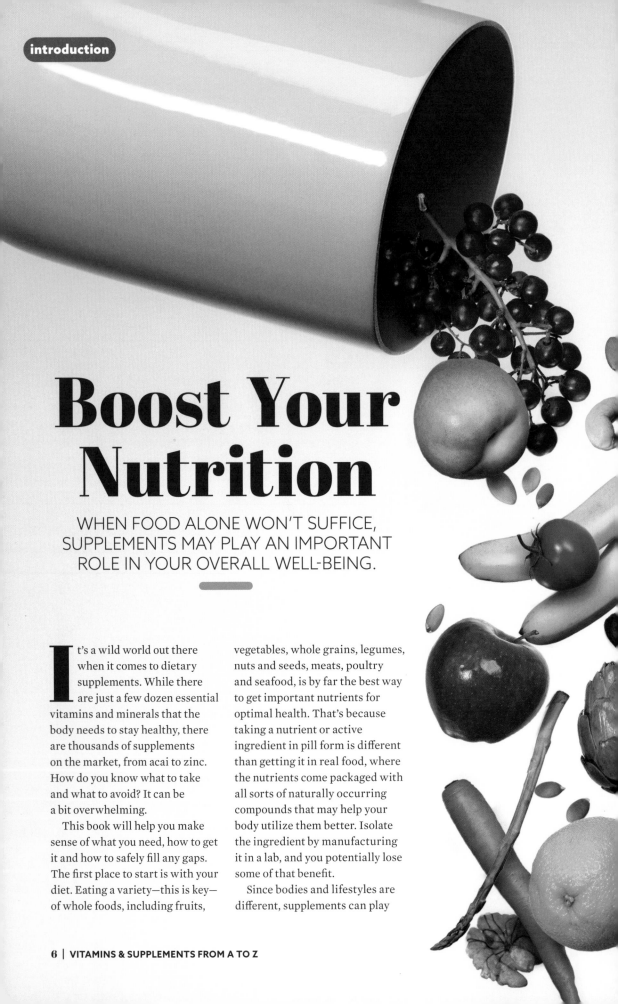

Boost Your Nutrition

WHEN FOOD ALONE WON'T SUFFICE,
SUPPLEMENTS MAY PLAY AN IMPORTANT
ROLE IN YOUR OVERALL WELL-BEING.

I t's a wild world out there when it comes to dietary supplements. While there are just a few dozen essential vitamins and minerals that the body needs to stay healthy, there are thousands of supplements on the market, from acai to zinc. How do you know what to take and what to avoid? It can be a bit overwhelming.

This book will help you make sense of what you need, how to get it and how to safely fill any gaps. The first place to start is with your diet. Eating a variety—this is key—of whole foods, including fruits,

vegetables, whole grains, legumes, nuts and seeds, meats, poultry and seafood, is by far the best way to get important nutrients for optimal health. That's because taking a nutrient or active ingredient in pill form is different than getting it in real food, where the nutrients come packaged with all sorts of naturally occurring compounds that may help your body utilize them better. Isolate the ingredient by manufacturing it in a lab, and you potentially lose some of that benefit.

Since bodies and lifestyles are different, supplements can play

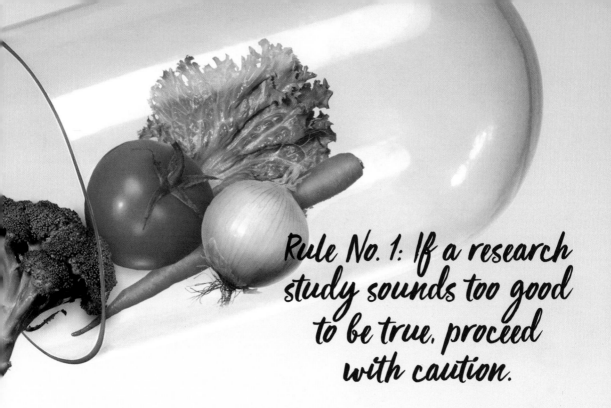

Rule No. 1: If a research study sounds too good to be true, proceed with caution.

an important role in shoring up gaps. If you're pregnant or trying to get pregnant, a senior, a smoker or have an underlying health condition, such as inflammatory bowel disease, you'll need to supplement certain nutrients. If you're an athlete or follow a restrictive diet, such as Paleo, keto or vegan, you may need to make up for some nutrient shortfalls. Food allergies, intolerances or sensitivities may also call for some supplementation, as can taking certain medications. This book is a good starting point, but your doctor and a qualified nutritionist can help you determine the best diet and supplementing strategy for your particular situation.

Buyer Beware

While there are established intake guidelines for essential vitamins and minerals, the same isn't true for herbal supplements, enzymes, probiotics and amino acids, which are a huge part of the market. It may take some experimenting to see what works. You don't

have to be a scientist to delve into the research, but you can develop some healthy skepticism. Most studies focus on a single standardized ingredient—calcium or SAM-e or ginseng—because it's easier to regulate the dosage and isolate the benefits of a single ingredient. If you scan store shelves, though, you'll find combination products, which might contain a few ingredients, such as melatonin, valerian and L-theanine. While each may have good research showing it can help improve sleep, it's harder to find independent data showing how all three work together. Who knows how the combination affects the mechanisms of action of each individual ingredient. The information in this book is focused on individual supplements only.

A good way to think about supplements is like any pill you might be prescribed. Don't take it if you don't need it, and start with the minimal effective dose.

While the FDA doesn't regulate supplement contents (but they do have a say in the claims that can be made on labels), they can have powerful effects. Always check the label or do your research on the manufacturer to make sure the product has been verified to contain what it's supposed to (this is a huge problem with supplements, especially those for weight loss, energy and libido).

Finally, taking handfuls of supplements forces your body to process and metabolize *all* their ingredients, including fillers—all the more reason to only take what you think you need. And while your body requires certain nutrients, such as calcium or vitamin E, for important functions, that doesn't mean more is better, especially since so many of our foods are already fortified with vitamins and minerals.

Read on to find out how to optimize your health, feel great and age better with the necessary nutrients.

MORE ISN'T ALWAYS BETTER WHEN IT COMES TO YOUR HEALTH.

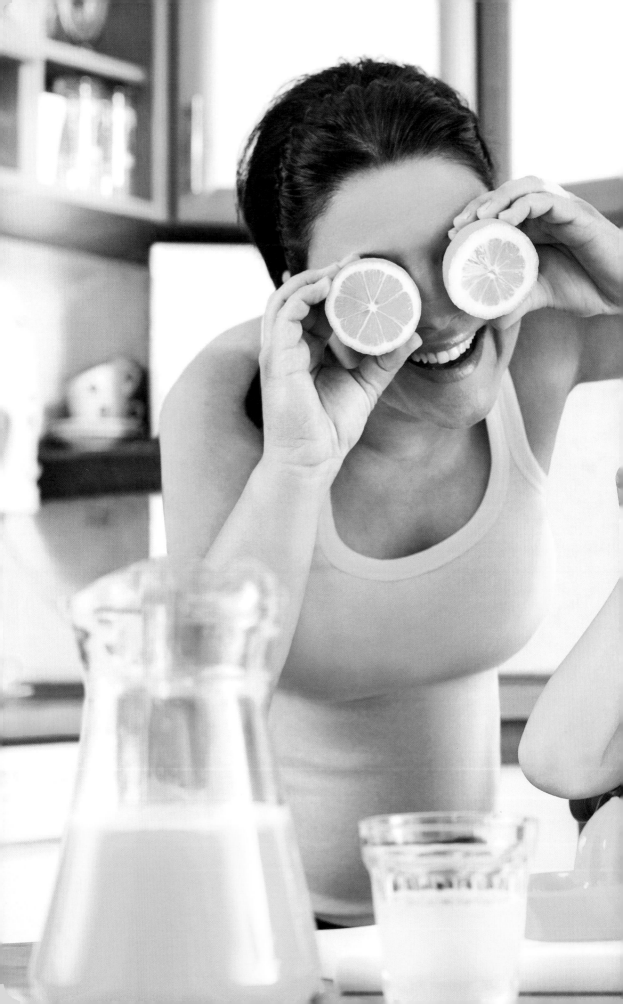

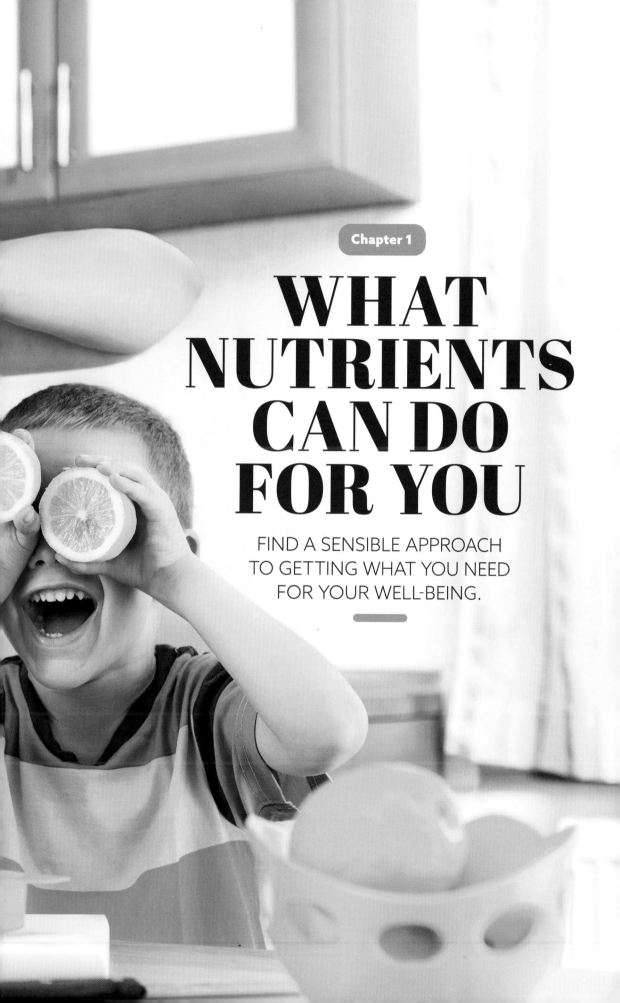

Chapter 1

WHAT NUTRIENTS CAN DO FOR YOU

FIND A SENSIBLE APPROACH
TO GETTING WHAT YOU NEED
FOR YOUR WELL-BEING.

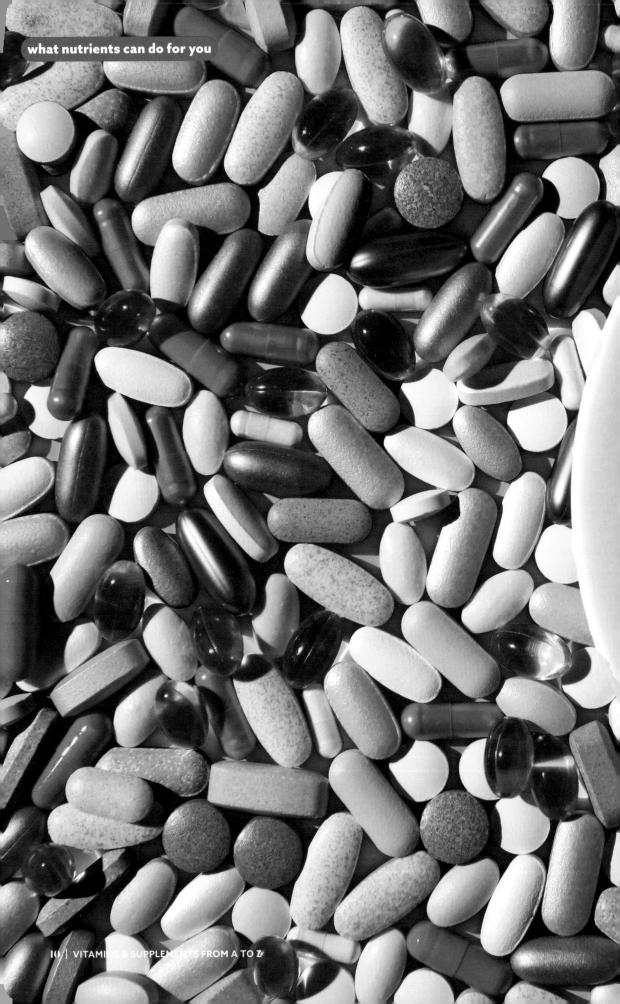

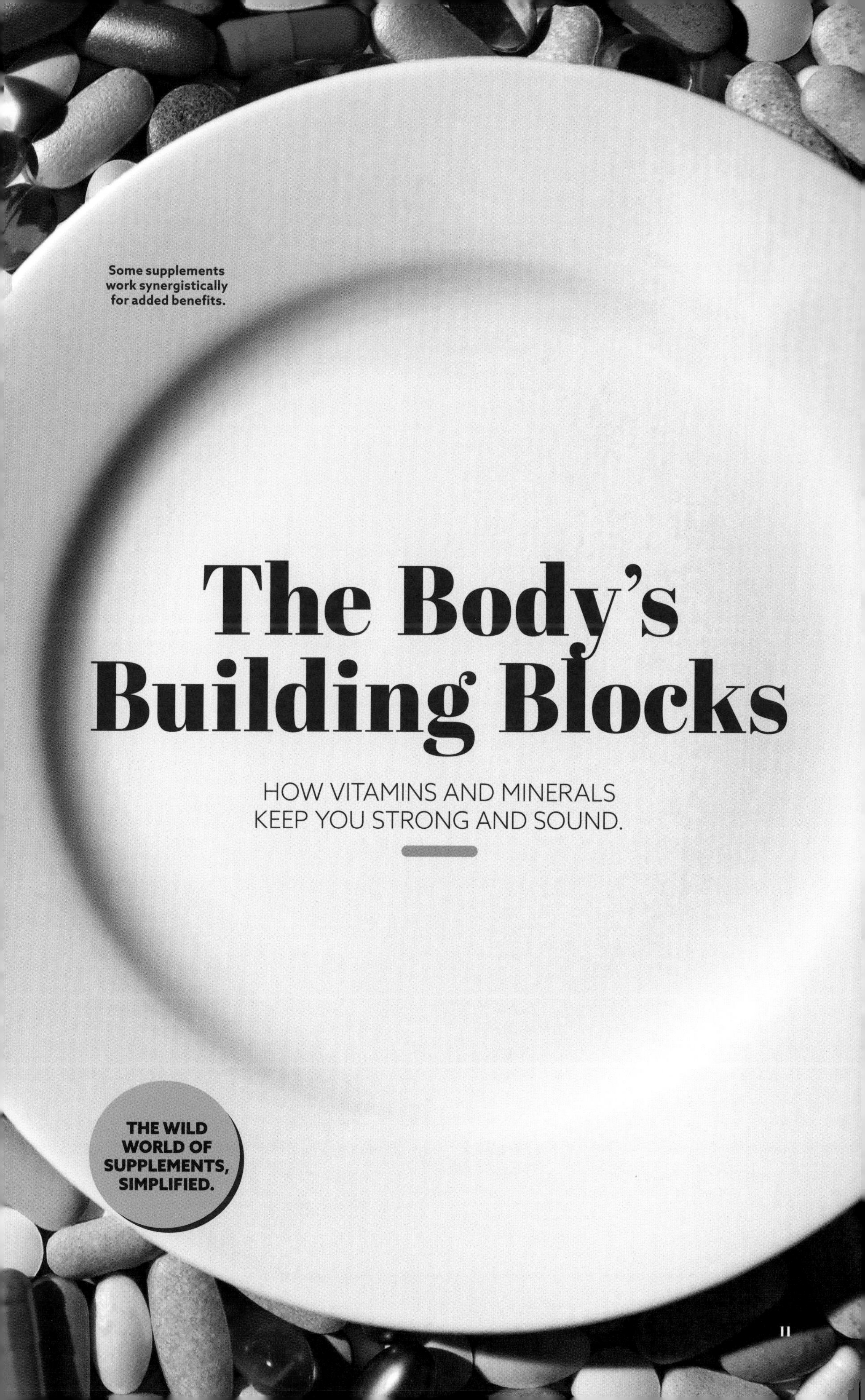

Some supplements
work synergistically
for added benefits.

The Body's Building Blocks

HOW VITAMINS AND MINERALS KEEP YOU STRONG AND SOUND.

**THE WILD
WORLD OF
SUPPLEMENTS,
SIMPLIFIED.**

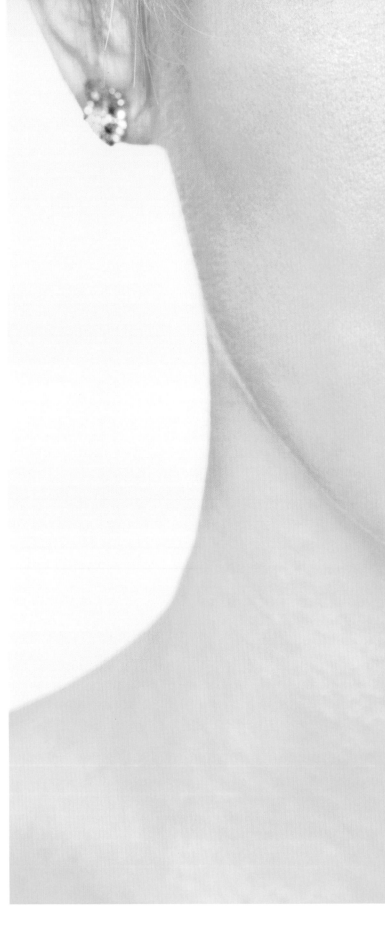

We spend a lot of time thinking about food, diet, carbohydrates, protein and fat. And while those aspects of eating are important, the vitamins, minerals and other nutrients we get from food are what keep the body, brain, muscles and organs functioning. Starting from the moment of conception, you're dependent on the nutrients you can glean from your mother's diet. Once you emerge, your nerves and brains cells must receive the proper vitamins in order to develop.

Throughout the rest of your life, you'll need a steady supply of vital nutrients to stay healthy, ward off disease and even keep your sanity. There are 13 essential vitamins, including vitamins A, C, D, E and K, and B vitamins such as riboflavin and folate. You also need minerals. And just like they sound, minerals are inorganic and found in soil and rocks. How do they make their way into your diet? Through plant foods, such as leafy greens and root vegetables, which absorb minerals from soil; meat also provides minerals because livestock absorb these essential nutrients from grazing on grass and grains.

Nutrient Nuts and Bolts

Drilling down deeper, there are two types of vitamins: fat-soluble and water-soluble. The fat-soluble vitamins are A, D, E and K, and they can take a little effort for the body to absorb. When you eat foods with fat—cooking oils, avocados, coconut, eggs—you get

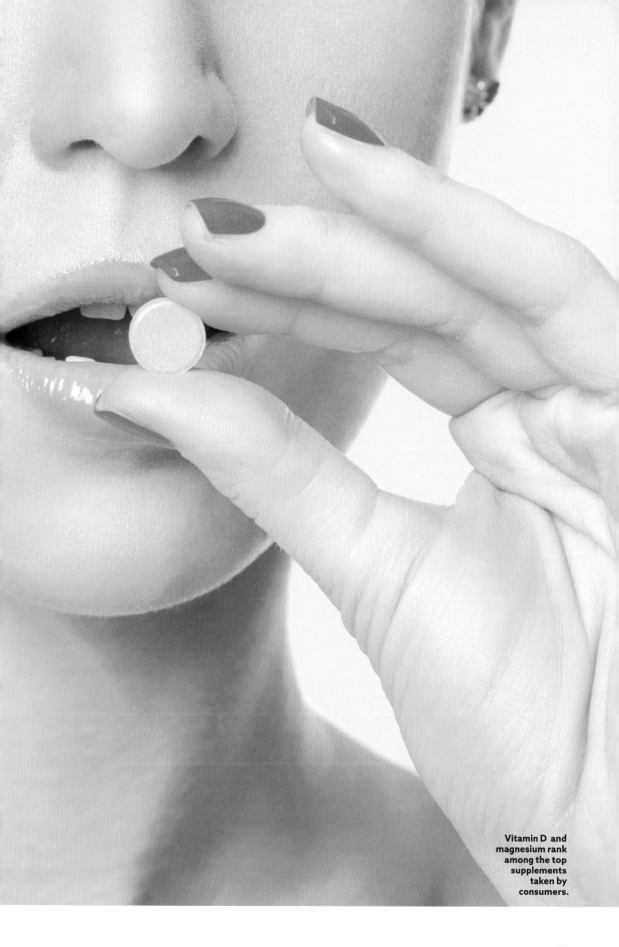

Vitamin D and magnesium rank among the top supplements taken by consumers.

fat-soluble vitamins. The bile in your small intestine breaks down the fats and absorbs the nutrients. They then bind with proteins and get put to use doing things such as helping build bone, protecting your eyes and assisting the body in absorbing other nutrients.

Any leftover fat-soluble vitamins get stored for later use in your liver and fat tissues. This means two things: You are less likely to fall deficient in fat-soluble vitamins, and it's

→ Six essential nutrients are carbohydrates, protein, fat, vitamins, minerals and water.

easier for these vitamins to build up in your body—potentially, to toxic levels.

All other vitamins are water-soluble—they arrive in your system from the fluid portions of the foods you eat—especially produce (which contains a lot of liquid). They're much easier to absorb, going straight from your digestive system into the bloodstream. Your kidneys monitor your levels of water-soluble vitamins and flush out any excess. This group of vitamins helps your body process energy from food and assists in the construction of proteins. They're also key to absorbing minerals.

Although most people believe any excess water-soluble vitamins are immediately flushed away, some are actually stored for a while. Vitamin B12 can stack up in your liver for years, although most of the rest will clear your system after—at most—a handful of days, which is why you have to eat those fruits and veggies every day.

Minerals also come in two categories—trace and macro. This distinction is pretty basic. You need only tiny amounts of trace minerals, so they're easy to get; you need more macrominerals. The trace minerals are iron, manganese, copper, iodine, zinc, cobalt, fluoride and selenium. Macrominerals include calcium, phosphorus, magnesium, sodium, potassium, chloride and sulfur. Some are quickly absorbed into the bloodstream in the same way water-soluble vitamins are; others—calcium, for example—require help from other nutrients to reach your bloodstream. Your body relies on minerals to keep your fluids balanced, and to replenish cells for your hair, nails, skin and skeleton.

With supplements, it's so easy to focus on treating illness and boosting energy that we forget the daily feats nutrients help achieve, including improving the following:

Your Metabolism

This is the process in your body that burns all the calories, and it involves digestion, energy, cell-building, breathing, heart rate and much more. The B vitamins are crucial to keeping your metabolism humming, according to the Mayo Clinic. They assist in converting carbs, protein and fat into energy, with a big assist from minerals such as magnesium.

Your Bones

This is where minerals can really shine. You know about calcium and bones, but magnesium and phosphorus also assist in the production of new bone, in addition to warding off fractures and osteoporosis. Vitamins such as D and K also come into play, because they help convert minerals into a substance the body can absorb.

Your Heart

While the nutrients that support metabolism also keep your heart ticking, some essential vitamins and minerals also reduce heart disease risk. Vitamins A, C and E function as antioxidants, which can calm inflammation. Vitamin B3 can help lower cholesterol, and minerals such as calcium, magnesium and potassium can keep blood pressure in check. All of this helps explain why a diet rich in produce helps your heart.

Your Life and Fertility

Without the right nutrients, you not only will be unlikely to conceive, but could also lose interest in sex altogether. Men need the mineral zinc to produce viable sperm and remain sexually active. Women planning on becoming pregnant need folic acid to protect the baby from birth defects. And both genders rely on vitamins C, E and B12 and the mineral selenium to keep in tip-top reproductive health.

All of this is a gentle reminder to make sure you stay up on your intake for *all* nutrients.

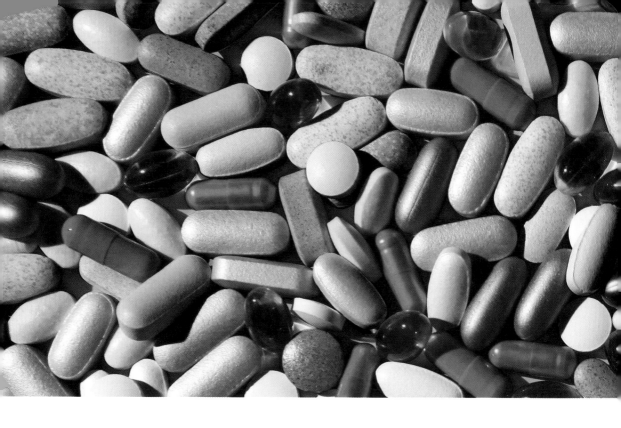

About half of all Americans
take a multivitamin.

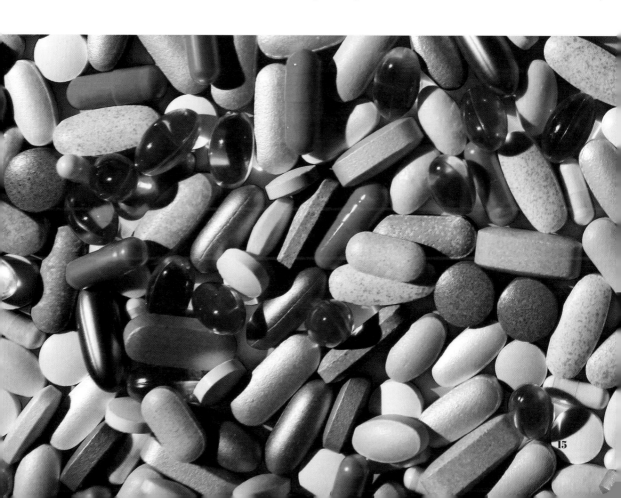

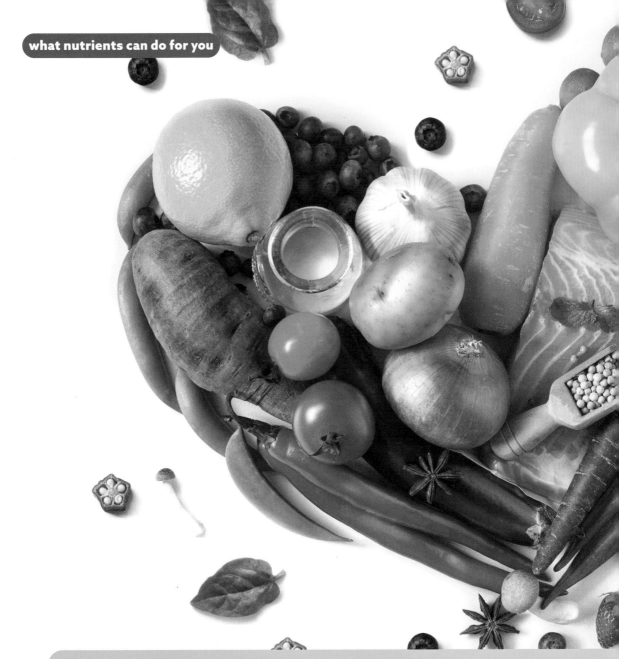

VITAMIN LINGO

Knowing a few phrases and acronyms will help you understand the jargon on the sides of pill bottles and potentially keep you safe.

RDA This is the Recommended Dietary Allowance established by the Institute of Medicine, in collaboration with other health agencies. RDAs indicate the average daily dietary intake of nutrients that a person needs to stay healthy. Backed by careful research, the RDAs are broken down by age and gender.

DRI To make things more complicated, the National Institutes of Health introduced Dietary Reference Intakes (which include RDAs) as a reference for what healthy people get of various minerals and vitamins. They're less prescriptive and more informational than RDAs.

AI Want one more measure? Try Adequate Intake—this is for nutrients that the government has yet to set an RDA or DRI for, but it wants to indicate

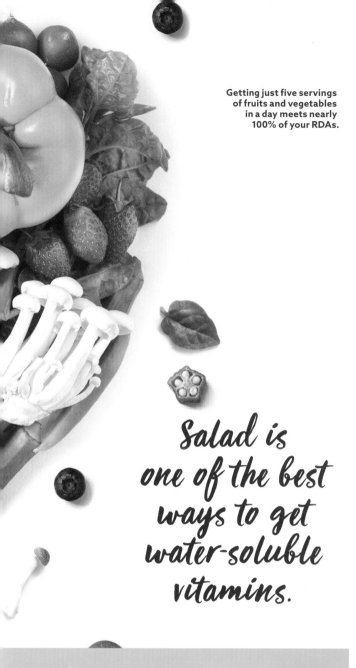

Getting just five servings of fruits and vegetables in a day meets nearly 100% of your RDAs.

Salad is one of the best ways to get water-soluble vitamins.

that the vitamin or mineral is probably important for good health.

UL And then there's the issue of how much is safe: The Upper Intake Level (UL) is the maximum tolerable amount that your body can handle before side effects kick in. Some of these symptoms can be subtle but deadly, so it's wise to respect this limit.

MEASUREMENT ABBREVIATIONS
You'll see a lot of different measurements on the sides of pill bottles, starting with mg (milligrams), which is usually next to vitamins and macrominerals. Trace nutrients are measured in micrograms (mcg). Often you'll see IU next to fat-soluble vitamins; it stands for international unit(s).

What About Antioxidants?

Every time someone starts talking about vitamins, it isn't too long before you hear the word *antioxidant*. Here's what that means.

Free Radicals// Whenever you're exposed to any form of toxin—air pollution, tobacco smoke, even sunlight—unstable molecules, known as free radicals, are created. They lack an electron, so they charge around, trying to steal one from other molecules— and wreak havoc in the process. Left to their own devices, free radicals damage tissues and can be the catalyst for serious illnesses such as heart disease and cancer.

Antioxidants// These compounds are able to give up an electron to stabilize free radicals. They come in all kinds of forms: vitamins, such as C and E; minerals (selenium is a well-known antioxidant); or compounds, like flavonoids (found in blueberries, onions and green tea) and carotenoids (which turn up in plums, kale and tomatoes).

In some cases, food is the best medicine.

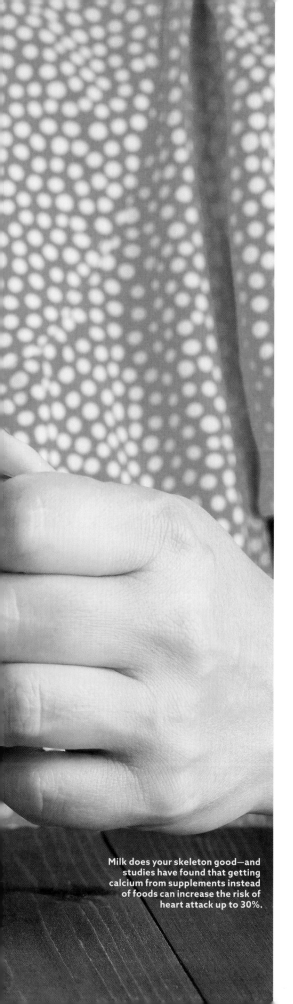

Milk does your skeleton good—and studies have found that getting calcium from supplements instead of foods can increase the risk of heart attack up to 30%.

EAT YOUR VITAMINS.

Stick to Food

THERE ARE SOME
VITAMINS AND MINERALS
YOU SHOULD PLAN
TO GET FROM YOUR DIET,
NOT THE DRUGSTORE.

—

A healthy eating plan is the best multivitamin you can have. And it tastes better!

Not all supplements are benign—or worth spending your hard-earned dollars on. If you eat a complete, well-rounded and healthy diet, there's a good chance you're covered for many of the most important nutrients. When people decide to take more of these vitamins and minerals in pill form, the water-soluble versions just get flushed through the digestive system. However, with some minerals and fat-soluble vitamins, the excess can build up to toxic levels, putting people at risk for some serious and even deadly conditions. There are always exceptions to the rules; but for the most part, these top-selling supplements are actually less effective than food sources.

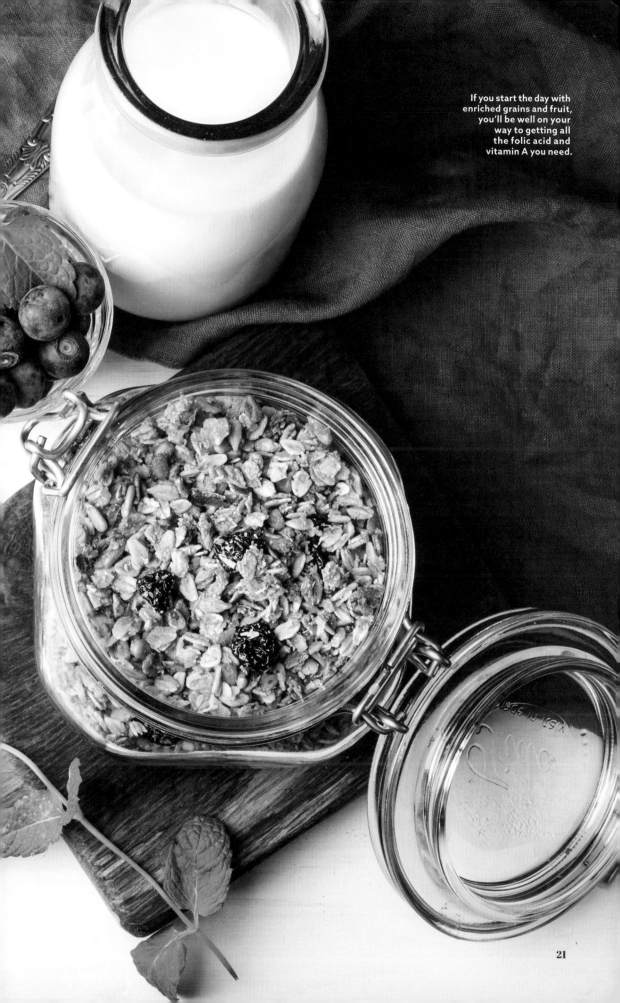

If you start the day with enriched grains and fruit, you'll be well on your way to getting all the folic acid and vitamin A you need.

21

Calcium

Calcium supplements get pushed on women as insurance for their bones. The notion is nice, but take note: Studies indicating that calcium protects against the bone-thinning disease osteoporosis have mostly looked at getting the mineral *from food*. Now, recent studies suggest that calcium supplements can raise the risk of kidney stones, high blood pressure and heart attack.

→ Not everything lives up to the sales pitch— especially when it comes to your health.

Researchers at the University of Iowa analyzed health information collected from 38,262 women over a seven-year period and found that those who were taking calcium supplements had a 17% higher risk of kidney stones. Calcium may also cause calcification in arteries, which has been tied to increases in blood pressure, says Stanley Goldfarb, MD, a professor of medicine at the University of Pennsylvania. In 2018, he wrote an editorial in the *Journal of Nephrology* that addressed the growing rate of complications from high levels of calcium.

Your daily calcium target should be between 1,000 and 1,300 mg a day, according to the National Institutes of Health. Take a look at your dietary sources: A cup of milk has 285 mg, and a cup of yogurt has 415 mg. A 1.5-ounce serving of cheese delivers between 300 and 450 mg. You also get calcium from dark, leafy greens such as spinach and kale (100–180 mg per ½ cup), canned sardines and pink salmon (with bones, 180–320 mg per 3 ounces), and soybeans (130 mg per ½ cup). What's more, calcium is the primary ingredient of many over-the-counter antacids. If you do take calcium in pills, stay vigilant, says Dr. Goldfarb: "Even at the recommended dose, yearly determinations of blood-calcium levels is a wise approach."

Folic Acid

This B vitamin is vital in preventing serious birth defects. Folic acid is so crucial to infant health that the government has mandated it be added to breakfast cereals and enriched grains. But if you take a multivitamin or supplement with 100% of the RDA for folic acid—400 micrograms (mcg)— your intake can start bumping up against the safe upper limit of 1,000 mcg. Harvard researchers theorized that a recent uptick in cases of colon cancer may be due to high levels of folic acid, although other studies dispute that claim. If you aren't pregnant or planning to conceive, you don't need to pop this extra pill.

Lycopene

This chemical pigment, found in red fruits and vegetables, appears to have antioxidant properties. Some studies suggest that lycopene may help guard against heart disease and several types of cancer, including breast, cervical, colon, kidney, lung, prostate and ovarian. It's even good for your eyesight—potentially protecting against cataracts.

However, it's important to know that all the studies have been on people who were eating lycopene in things such as pink grapefruit, watermelon and tomatoes—especially cooked tomatoes. Cooking transforms lycopene into a more easily digestible form, which is why foods that contain cooked tomatoes—think sauces, pastas, even ketchup—are your best bet.

Omega-3 Fatty Acids

Omega-3 fatty acids have long been thought to help lower the risk of heart disease, but taking the supplement form can leave a fishy taste in your mouth. A 2020 study published in the *American Journal of Clinical Nutrition* shows that consuming walnuts may be the way to go. Scientists discovered a walnut-enriched diet protects the heart, and may improve memory.

Vitamin A

You can get vitamin A in several forms. The retinol form,

from animal sources such as eggs and whole milk, is more readily absorbed than the other type—beta-carotene. But even vegetarians can meet their needs by eating five servings a day of produce such as dark, leafy greens and orange and yellow fruits.

Taking vitamin A supplements can pose issues—too much retinol can cause birth defects and liver abnormalities, and it might harm bones. Researchers have found that people who take high doses of beta-carotene supplements have a higher risk of cancer and heart disease. Beta-carotene works well when you get it from colorful foods such as spinach, yams and bell peppers.

Vitamin E

Vitamin E is a powerful antioxidant that protects cells from the harmful molecules known as free radicals. It's important for immunity, healthy blood vessel function and clotting. But when taken as a supplement, it's also potentially dangerous. Two analyses of vitamin E research have linked as little as 400 IU a day to a small but significant increase in the risk of premature death. Because vitamin E can interfere with blood clotting, it shouldn't be taken with blood thinners. And while wheat-germ oil packs more vitamin E than any other food source, you might find it easier to get the nutrient from sunflower seeds or almonds; an ounce of each packs about a third of your daily requirement.

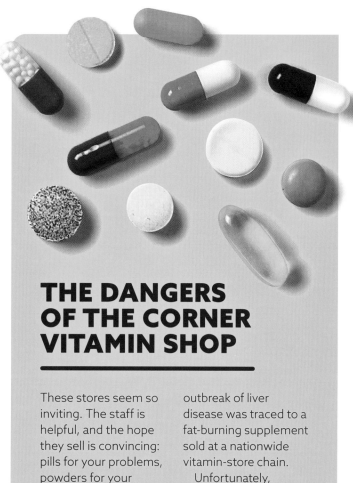

THE DANGERS OF THE CORNER VITAMIN SHOP

These stores seem so inviting. The staff is helpful, and the hope they sell is convincing: pills for your problems, powders for your muscles, herbs for your ailments. But proceed with caution. Supplements are loosely regulated, and all kinds of unpleasant surprises turn up in seemingly innocent pills all the time.

A study from the U.S. Food and Drug Administration found that many weight-loss and workout supplements contained chemicals similar to amphetamine—a serious and potentially dangerous stimulant.

In another troubling case, a multistate outbreak of liver disease was traced to a fat-burning supplement sold at a nationwide vitamin-store chain.

Unfortunately, dietary supplements account for nearly 20% of drug-related liver injuries in the emergency room, according to the Centers for Disease Control and Prevention (CDC). If you want to be safe, don't be swayed by the in-store sales pitch. Talk with your doctor about what you might need, and consider getting tested for any potential shortfalls in nutrients. (See "Should You Get Your Nutrient Levels Checked?" on page 35.)

New moms and folks
over 50 are among the people
who need extra nutrients.

Who Really Needs Supplements?

IF YOU FALL INTO ONE OF THE FOLLOWING CATEGORIES, YOU DO.

A lthough plenty of people could probably benefit from taking a multivitamin to help make up for a weak diet—or the foods they just won't eat (looking at you, fish haters), there are certain groups who just can't get what they need, no matter how well they eat. Definitely discuss your options with your doctor first, but make sure that you're covering your needs. Here are the conditions that demand you take a supplement—and what to do about it.

People on low-calorie diets often miss out on nutrients.

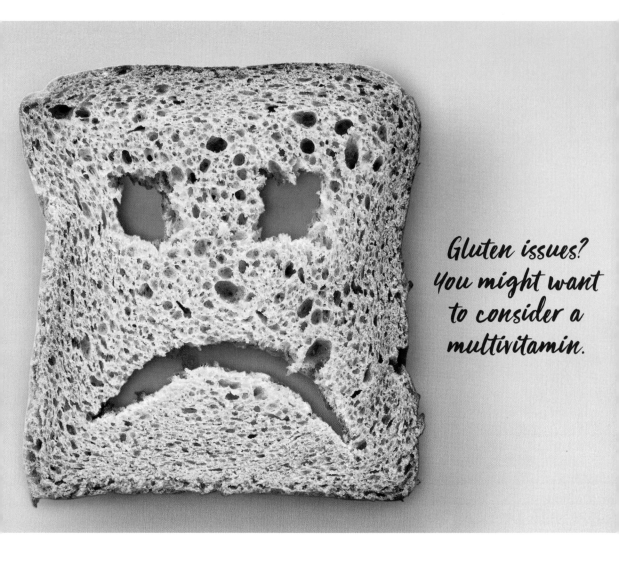

Gluten issues? You might want to consider a multivitamin.

You're Pregnant or Breastfeeding

It's not just for you, but also for your baby. For example, folic acid can help prevent a type of birth defect that affects the brain and spinal cord. Calcium is for mom: It can help maintain bone density while the developing fetus is building its own skeleton. Iodine is crucial for keeping mom's thyroid in working order, because a deficiency could stunt the baby's growth and cause mental disability. Finally, making sure mom is up on her iron will ensure enough oxygen for baby. A typical prenatal vitamin might include:

- *400 mcg folic acid*
- *400 IU vitamin D*
- *200 to 300 mg calcium*
- *70 mg vitamin C*
- *3 mg thiamine*
- *2 mg riboflavin*
- *20 mg niacin*
- *6 mcg vitamin B12*
- *10 mg vitamin E*
- *15 mg zinc*
- *17 mg iron*
- *150 mcg iodine*

Many breastfeeding moms will continue with their prenatal vitamin, though it may contain more iron than they need, according to experts at the University of California, San Francisco. If you struggle with stomach upset or constipation, you can switch to a multivitamin with 100% of the RDA for iron.

You're a Vegan or a Vegetarian

Despite how healthy these dietary choices are, vegans and some types of vegetarians can miss out

→ Poor nutrition during pregnancy can lead to health issues for the baby.

on important nutrients. These include vitamin B12, which mostly comes from meat, and vitamin D, which is in fortified dairy—although the body can make it when your skin is exposed to sunlight. Iodine and calcium—which dairy can supply—may also be issues, and you can fall short on iron and zinc, depending on the type of diet you follow. Consider these options:

- 25–100 mcg/day vitamin B12
- 1,000 IU/day vitamin D
- 90 mcg/day iodine (or make sure you use iodized salt—sparingly)
- Calcium, iron, zinc: Check with your doctor before supplementing.

You're on a Low-Calorie Diet

Generally, low-calorie diet plans aren't a great idea: People usually gain the weight back quickly once they start eating normally again. But if you're following one, consider a multivitamin, because you'll be missing out on nutrients that your body desperately needs. And you should consider a more sustainable weight-loss plan.

You're a Picky Eater

If you or your kids are extremely picky eaters, you may want to add a multivitamin. Talk to your pediatrician about children's needs and what type of supplement would best fill the gap.

You Have Food Allergies

Depending on the type of allergy, you can end up short on calcium (milk); iron and B vitamins (eggs); riboflavin, vitamin B6 and zinc (soy). Luckily, it's possible to make up the difference with other foods—beef, fish and poultry can add back a lot of necessary nutrients; fortified foods such as breakfast cereals can also help. Talk to your doctor or a registered dietitian about smart ways to supplement for your allergy.

You Have Celiac Disease

People with undiagnosed celiac disease are nutrient-deficient across the board, because the body isn't able to glean all the health-sustaining goodness from the foods they eat. But even after taking steps to eliminate gluten from their diet, celiac sufferers can still wind up short on folate, vitamin B12 and magnesium, according to research published in the *Annals of Medicine*. You may also need to take calcium and vitamin D to help shore up your bones. You can also try dietary supplements that may help relieve your symptoms. Aim for 100% of the RDA for these nutrients.

You're on Certain Medications

If you're taking drugs to lower your cholesterol, blood pressure

THE DEETS

When shopping for supplements, stick with familiar, established brands—or ask a pharmacist or registered dietitian for recommendations. Also consider the following:

Check the Label for Certification// Consumerlab.com and United States Pharmacopeia (USP) offer a stamp of approval if a manufacturer meets basic standards and passes third-party testing.

Read the Claims// Sexual aids, weight-loss pills and energy-boosting potions are the most likely to be adulterated with substances that could cause trouble.

Avoid "Kitchen-Sink" Pills// A multivitamin that also contains herbs and other supposed "wonder" substances is more likely to contain potentially dangerous mystery ingredients; they may also interact with other drugs you're taking.

27

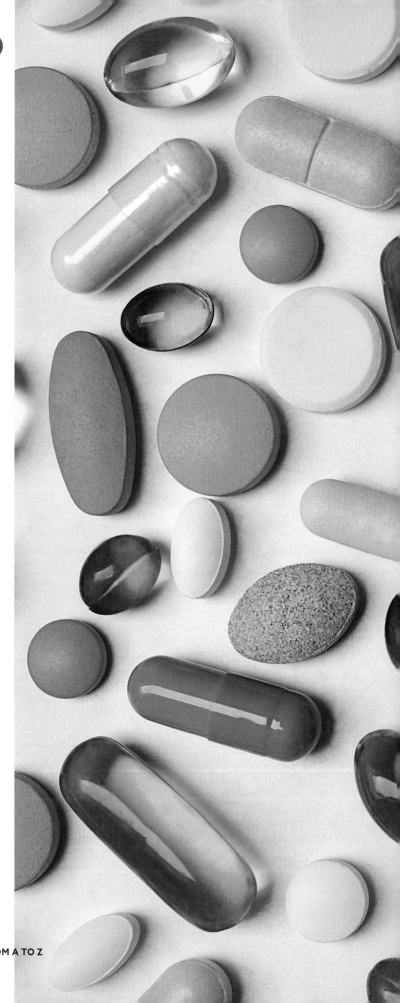

Check with your doc to avoid potential Rx interactions.

or stomach acid (due to stomach upset), you could be low in B12, folic acid or fat-soluble vitamins such as A, D, E and K. Why? Those drugs can interfere with your body's ability to absorb these nutrients. Depending on how long you'll be on the medication, you will want to discuss supplementing your diet with your physician.

You're Over 50

As you age, your body becomes less efficient at extracting and absorbing nutrients. Eating more nutrient-dense foods, such as richly colored fruits and vegetables, can help, although nutrition experts now recommend that this age group also take 100 mcg of vitamin B12 daily. Deficiency in B12 is linked to depression, confusion, balance issues, memory problems and even dementia.

Consider regularly visiting your doctor to have your vitamin levels tested, so you can address any potential deficiencies. (See "Should You Get Your Nutrient Levels Checked?" on page 35.)

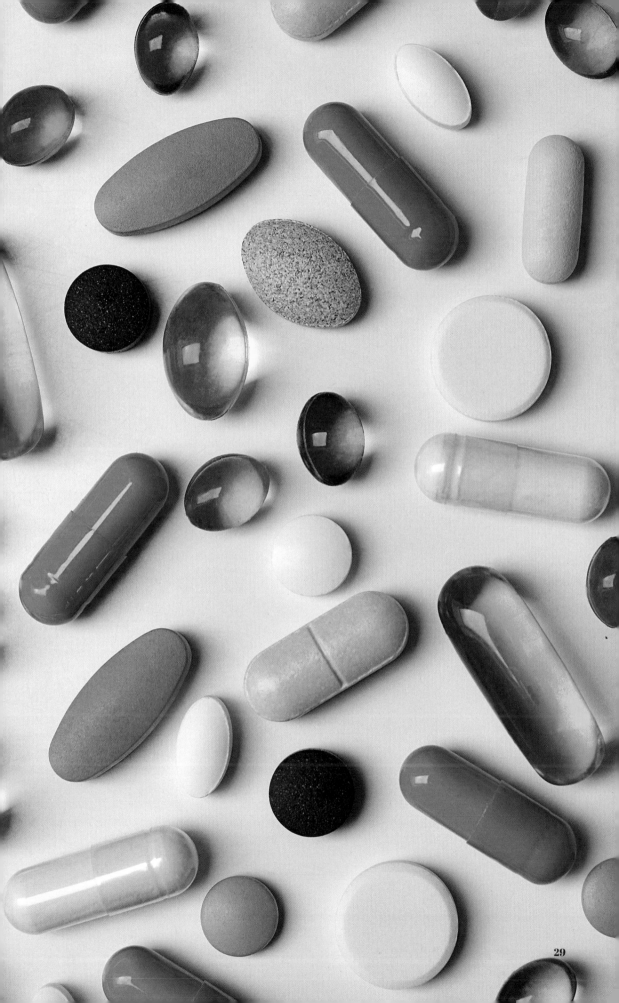

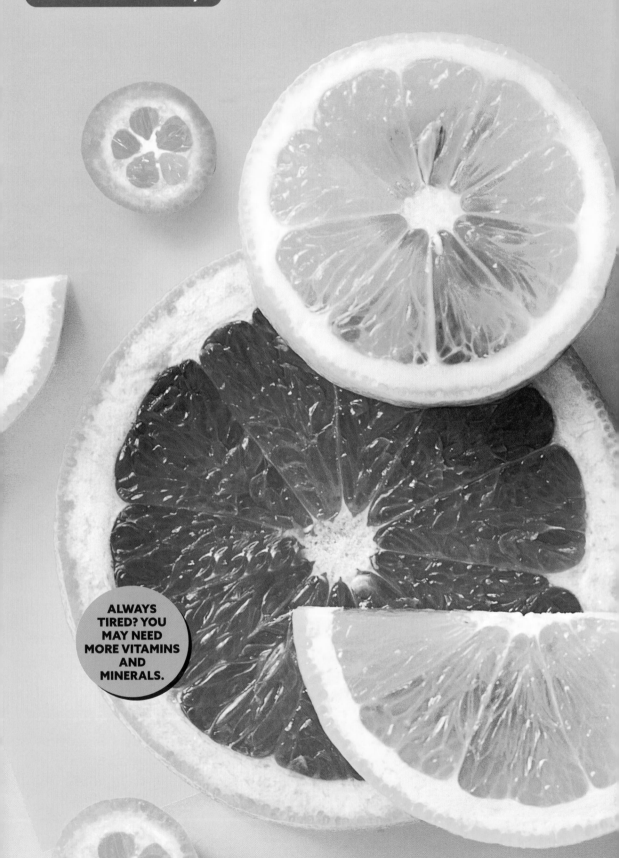

ALWAYS TIRED? YOU MAY NEED MORE VITAMINS AND MINERALS.

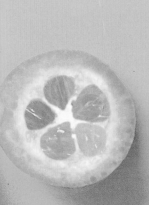

The Most Common Deficiencies

BEWARE OF THESE SYMPTOMS—YOU COULD BE DANGEROUSLY SHORT ON KEY NUTRIENTS.

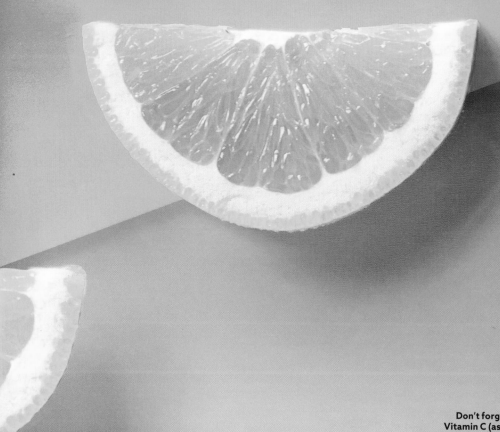

Don't forget your citrus! Vitamin C (ascorbic acid) is necessary for the growth, development and repair of all body tissues and is involved in collagen production, iron absorption, wound healing, and the maintenance of cartilage, bones and teeth.

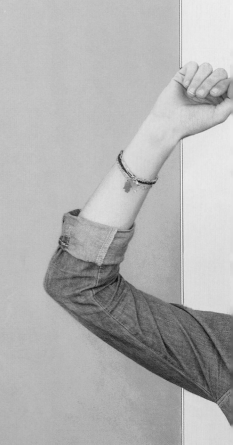

Correct your nutrient shortfalls to feel amazing!

When you can buy perfect mangoes in January and get nearly farm-fresh kale year-round, it's hard to believe that anyone might end up falling short on nutrients—but it happens, according to the Centers for Disease Control and Prevention (CDC). In the agency's findings, nearly 10% of Americans fall short—and that's not even counting those among us who could benefit from getting *more* than the recommended daily amounts of certain vitamins and minerals.

Depending on where you live, the soil may be deficient in vital minerals, leaving you low; or your geographic location could mean that, for much of the year, you're deprived of enough sun to naturally produce nutrients that your heart, bones and metabolism depend upon.

Following are the symptoms that may indicate you need a supplement. The nutrients listed include those we commonly miss

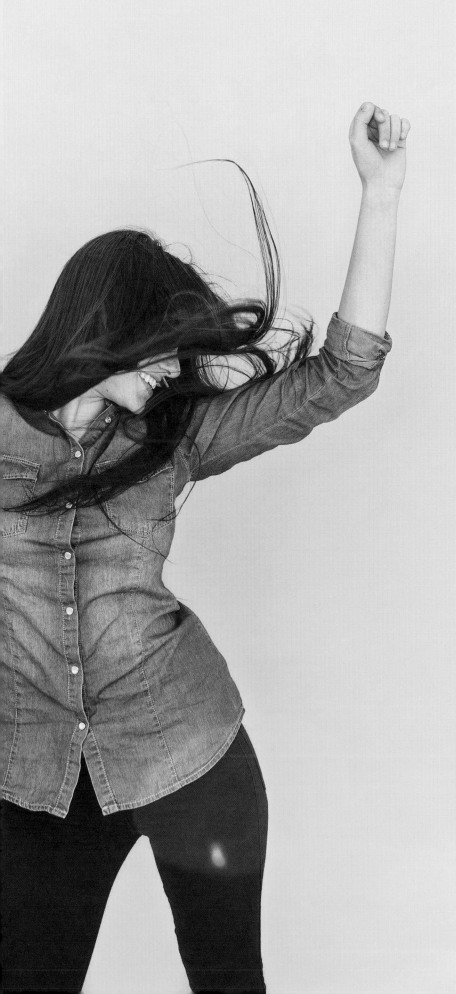

Want to feel fantastic? Grab some vitamin B to get a boost of energy.

out on, as well as some that we could probably use more of for better protection from deadly and chronic diseases. But before you self-diagnose, talk to your doctor about your diet and your nutritional needs.

→ As you age, your body won't absorb nutrients as well. You'll likely need a supplement to keep up.

SYMPTOMS

Fatigue; Muddy Thinking; Feeling Cold; Enlarged Thyroid Gland

DEFICIENCY

Iodine//

We tend to take this trace element for granted. Table salt is fortified with iodine, so we all get plenty, right? That all depends: In this day of gourmet Celtic, smoked and Hawaiian salts, plus recipes that increasingly call for kosher salt, people are getting much less ordinary table salt—the primary source of iodine in the diet. According to the American Thyroid Association, iodine intake in the U.S. dropped by half between the 1970s and the 2000s. While as a nation we're still comfortably above the 150 mcg a day most adults need, the decline of iodized salt use brings with it the real possibility that some of us are falling into deficiency.

Why is iodine important? Because of your thyroid—a butterfly-shaped gland in your neck. It helps regulate your heart rate, your metabolism and numerous other vital body functions through the release of signaling hormones. The only way your thyroid is able to produce these hormones is with the help of iodine. When its levels fall, the thyroid senses a hormone shortage and begins working overtime to generate more. Eventually the strain can cause the thyroid to swell into a neck goiter, but other problems occur well in advance of visible changes. People with a mild iodine deficiency can experience fatigue, depression and weight gain. And in children, a lack of iodine can stall brain and nerve development, potentially lowering IQ and stunting growth.

To be sure you get enough, keep iodized table salt for baking (where it works better than slower-to-dissolve gourmet salts) and in the shaker. You won't need much—a teaspoon of fortified salt delivers 400 mcg of iodine. You can also get iodine from eggs, dairy, fish, shellfish and the kelp used to wrap sushi.

SYMPTOMS

Light-Headedness; Fast Heart Rate; Palpitations; Brittle Nails; Shortness of Breath

DEFICIENCY

Iron//

The most common nutrient deficiency worldwide is a lack of iron. The mineral plays a key role in distributing oxygen to muscles and other tissues throughout the body; it also supports your immune system, helping ward off infection. When your iron levels fall, the resulting lack of energy can keep you from engaging in the physical activity you need to help maintain your health and weight.

The trick is that even if you're getting enough iron, other nutrients and drugs can inhibit your body's ability to absorb this vital nutrient. Do you take calcium pills? They can block the absorption of iron. So can antacids, the antibiotic neomycin and the blood-thinning drug warfarin. For women, heavy periods, pregnancy and breastfeeding all increase the need for the nutrient. Just growing older can deplete iron levels, because the stomach acid you need to digest iron decreases as you age.

Supplements are an option, but be careful and make sure to discuss with your doctor: Getting too much iron can be deadly. Adult men need about 8 mg a day; adult women need at least 18 mg. You can get plenty from a healthy diet. Good sources include organ meats such as liver, which has around 6 mg a serving. Lean cuts of red meat provide about 2.5 mg a serving. For plant sources, try beans (2 to 3 mg), asparagus, chard or spinach (3 to 4 mg), and spices such as turmeric, thyme or cumin (1 mg per teaspoon). Note that your body will be able to squeeze more iron from plant sources if you pair them with vitamin C–rich foods such as citrus fruits, peppers, broccoli or tomatoes.

Confusion;
Irritability;
Muscle Pain

DEFICIENCY

Vitamin B6 (Pyridoxine)//

This is the nutrient Americans are most likely to be deficient in, according to the CDC. Vitamin B6 is crucial to healthy brain development in children and to maintain the integrity of your nervous and immune systems. It also helps make hemoglobin, which delivers oxygen to organs and muscles.

People fall short when they have digestive disorders such as celiac, Crohn's or inflammatory bowel disease; patients with kidney issues can also have trouble absorbing the nutrient. As we age, the recommended daily allowance of B6 increases, and getting enough may help prevent heart disease, certain types of cancer and even dementia. For pregnant women, there's evidence that low levels of B6 may contribute to morning sickness.

Adults need between 1.3 mg and 1.7 mg a day; good food sources include chickpeas (1.1 mg per serving), tuna (0.9 mg), fortified breakfast cereals (0.5 mg) and bananas (0.5 mg).

SYMPTOMS

Muscle Pain;
Fatigue; Weakness

DEFICIENCY

Vitamin D//

You've probably heard of the so-called "sunshine vitamin"— vitamin D—and how important it is for healthy bones and possible protection against cancer (a new study reveals high levels may lower the risk for breast cancer), heart disease and other chronic conditions. Yet so many people fail to get enough of this vital nutrient that the Endocrine Society—a national group dedicated to research on hormones, metabolism and bone health—is now calling for at-risk populations to get their vitamin D levels tested—and people who are overweight are the most at-risk.

Falling short on vitamin D is easy: For much of the year, Americans who live north of a line that stretches from New York City to Portland, Oregon, typically don't get enough sunlight for their bodies to generate the nutrient (sunlight is the most common source). The elderly can suffer deficiencies because the body's vitamin D–making machinery breaks down with age. Other at-risk populations include children; pregnant and nursing women; anyone who is dark-skinned; and people with digestive disorders, such as inflammatory bowel disease.

SHOULD YOU GET YOUR NUTRIENT LEVELS CHECKED?

That's a discussion to have with your primary care physician: If you eat a healthy diet and feel fine, there's little reason to get tested. However, for some people with genetic conditions or who live in northern climes, testing for specific nutrient deficiencies—like vitamin D—may make sense.

Some tests that screen for a wide range of nutrient deficiencies include: SpectraCell, Walk-In-Lab and Nutritionally Yours. If vitamin D is a specific concern, you can ask your doctor about the test offered by the Vitamin D Council (although the other screens can do individual nutrient testing as well).

You order the test through your doctor— or a nearby lab that offers the tests—and have your blood drawn there. Or you can order a kit through the mail and then go to a local clinic to have the blood drawn; some tests offer a finger-prick device so you can collect the blood at home.

The results will indicate whether your levels are adequate or deficient, and the lab may offer recommendations for making up any shortfalls. Always discuss a plan of action with your doctor first to make sure you don't overdo it or take something that might interfere with your other medications.

Following a healthy lifestyle helps save money by eliminating the need for multivitamins.

And, for reasons that aren't completely clear, the obese are also deficient. One explanation is that vitamin D gets trapped in fat cells—so losing weight helps release those stores of D, automatically raising levels. Anyone who falls into any of these groups should talk to their doctor about getting a test for their vitamin D levels. (Government health officials recommend you get between 400 and 800 IU daily, depending on your age.)

Before you apply sunscreen, say government health officials, let your forearms and face soak in 10 to 15 minutes of sun two to three days a week (avoid between the hours of 10-4, when harmful UV is strongest). You can also get D from fortified eggs, milk and soy products; button mushrooms; and oily fish such as salmon, sardines and oysters.

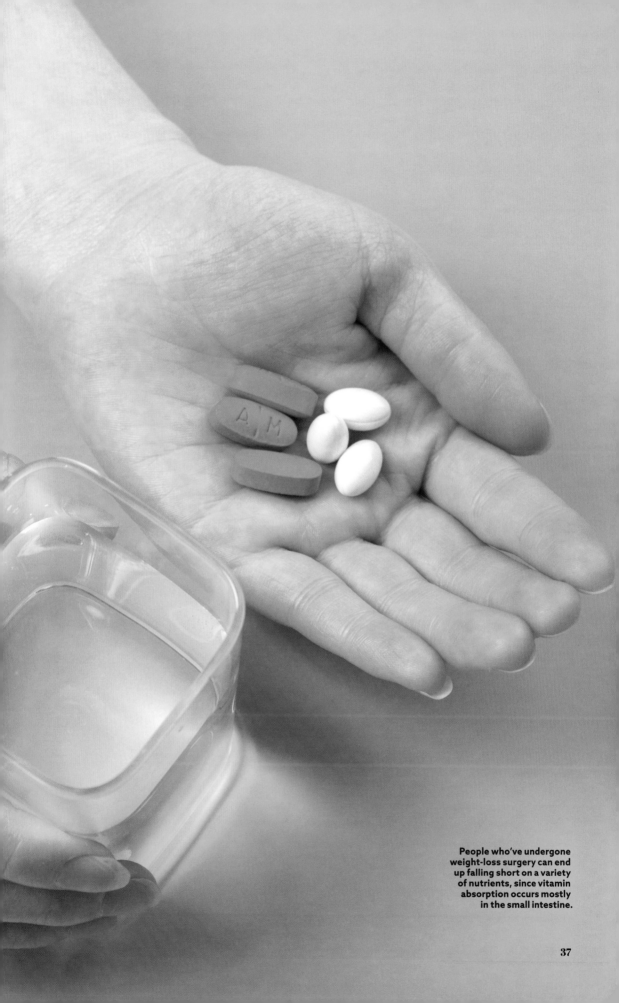

People who've undergone weight-loss surgery can end up falling short on a variety of nutrients, since vitamin absorption occurs mostly in the small intestine.

Take your multivitamin and any B vitamins in the morning, when your body best absorbs the nutrients and so they won't interfere with sleep or be overstimulating.

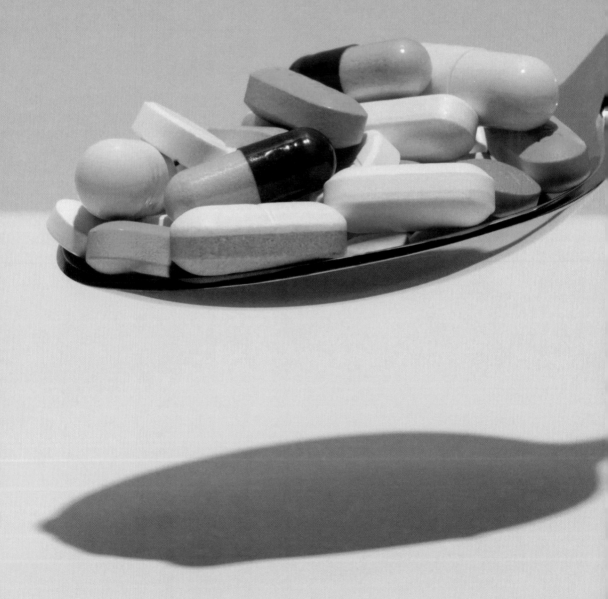

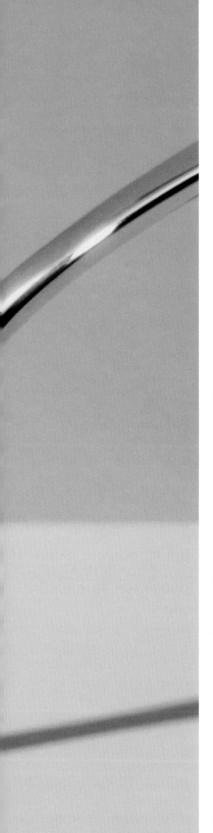

Every cell in your body requires magnesium to function—it's involved in more than 300 reactions, from creating new proteins to repairing DNA.

SYMPTOMS

Muscle Twitches
and Cramps;
Irregular Heartbeat;
Difficulty Breathing

DEFICIENCY

Magnesium//
This mineral plays a role in more than 300 biochemical reactions in your body, supporting immunity, keeping your heart rate regular, promoting healthy blood pressure and helping build strong bones. Magnesium even facilitates the conversion of carbohydrates and fat into energy for your muscles, meaning that getting enough will help you maintain your weight and your get-up-and-go.

And there's more: Researchers at the Karolinska Institute in Stockholm have found that a 100 mg daily decrease in magnesium is linked to a 10% increase in stroke risk. To arrive at their results, the Swedish researchers pooled the results of seven separate studies that involved nearly 250,000 people and nearly 6,500 cases of stroke.

The results are unsettling, because in the United States, the average magnesium intake of men (320 mg a day) and women (230 mg a day) is about 100 mg lower than what the government recommends (420 mg and 320 mg, respectively).

What's the best way to get more magnesium? You can take a supplement, although you should discuss that with a doctor or dietitian first. They will recommend getting more from your diet, such as leafy green vegetables (80 mg a serving), beans (50–80 mg; white or navy beans have 96 mg), nuts (60–75 mg), whole-grain cereals (check the label) and pumpkin seeds (about 120 mg).

THERE IS NO REPLACEMENT FOR HEALTHY EATING.

Get your nutrition
from food first.

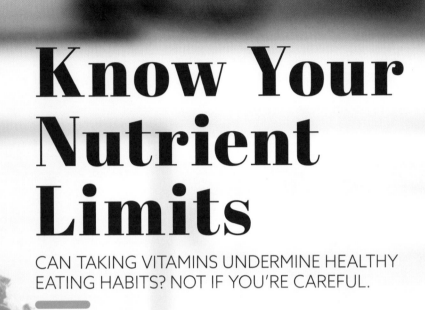

Know Your Nutrient Limits

CAN TAKING VITAMINS UNDERMINE HEALTHY
EATING HABITS? NOT IF YOU'RE CAREFUL.

DON'T
LET A
MULTIVITAMIN
WRECK
YOUR DIET.

We tend to look to multivitamins and other supplements as ways to balance a poor diet. People believe that this insurance-policy approach to nutrition can make up for missing out on servings of produce or indulging in fast food for lunch. And while this kind of "umbrella coverage" can help fill in nutrients that you might be missing from your diet, depending on it could leave your health exposed—even undermined.

A False Sense of Security

"People who rely on dietary-supplement use for health protection may pay a hidden price: the curse of licensed self-indulgence," says Wen-Bin Chiou, MD, a nutrition researcher and professor at Taiwan's National Sun Yat-sen University, author of a study on just this phenomenon.

Dr. Chiou and colleagues gave volunteers a multivitamin or a placebo and—in a twist—let them know which was which, when in fact *all* the pills were placebos. They then had the volunteers fill out questionnaires on the desirability of various behaviors, ranging from healthy (running, yoga, swimming) to hedonistic (sunbathing, excessive drinking, casual sex). People who believed they had taken a multivitamin rated the hedonistic activities as much more desirable than members of the placebo group, who were more likely to rank healthy behaviors as desirable.

After the questionnaires were filled out, the researchers offered the volunteers lunch coupons that would pay for a buffet or an organic meal. The multivitamin group shunned the organic meal in favor of the buffet, even though they perceived the organic meal as healthier. The placebo group was more likely to choose the organic lunch. Chiou believes it's clear that the healthy behavior of swallowing a vitamin led that group to give themselves license when it came to less-healthy behavior. Conversely, the people who knew that they got a placebo were more likely to make some healthier decisions.

In a second test, Chiou pulled off the same subterfuge of giving a fake multivitamin or a placebo to volunteers. He then asked the participants to test a pedometer for research purposes, instructing them to walk to either of two different landmarks. Both groups were given an hour to complete the task and were encouraged to run errands or visit a friend along the way. More than two-thirds of the multivitamin-takers chose the closer landmark, compared to just 40% of the placebo group. What's more, the placebo group also covered more distance, on average, than those who had taken the faux multivitamin. The results suggest that people may subconsciously believe the pills give them an excuse to bend or even break the rules of healthy living, says Chiou.

THE DEETS

Fortification

Ever notice how some breakfast cereals deliver nearly 100% of your RDAs? Or that milk contains vitamin D? That's fortification, and it's helped Americans avoid health issues such as rickets, osteoporosis and goiters. However...

Avoid Over-Supplementing//
Because we get so many nutrients from fortified foods, taking supplements blindly can easily push you past safe limits.

Talk to an Expert//
If you're interested in supplementing your diet, sit down and have a chat with your doctor or a registered dietitian (RD). You'll get a better sense of what is best for you.

KNOW YOUR NUTRIENT NEEDS BEFORE YOU DIVE IN.

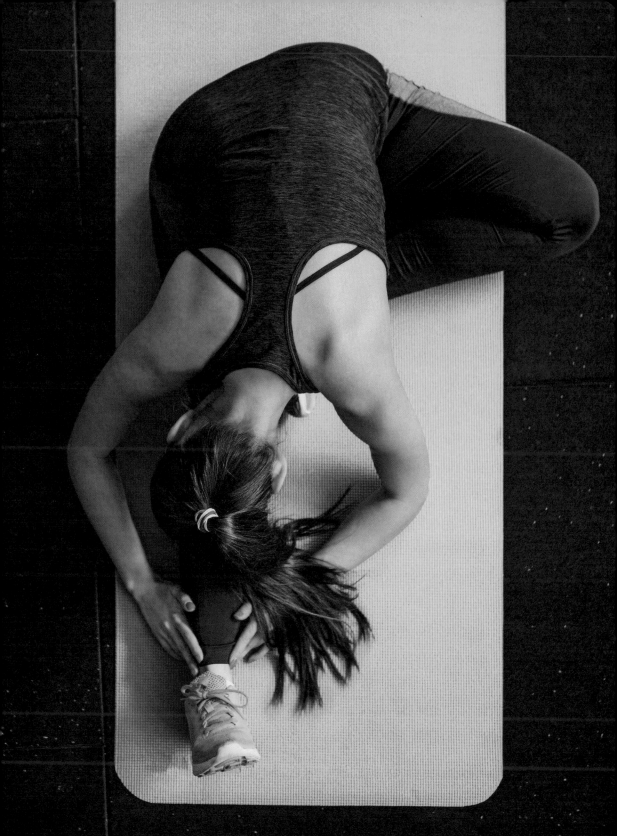

Eating a healthy diet may be better than taking multivitamins.

Only 1 in 10 U.S. adults get enough fruit and vegetables in their diet.

Many phytochemicals come straight from fresh foods.

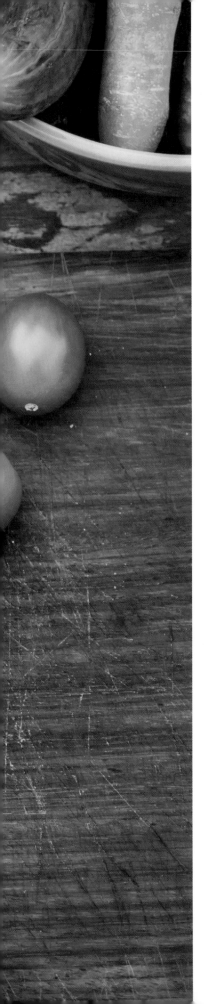

The Truth About Multivitamins

Recent studies have stipulated that taking a multivitamin is likely a waste of money for most people. The theory: They may not have a significant impact on your risk of heart disease, stroke or death from any cause and can give a false sense of security. Most nutrition experts point to studies in which regular vitamin-takers do no better—or even worse—than people who skip supplements. In fact, research published in the *Archives of Internal Medicine* found that elderly women who regularly took multivitamins had a higher risk of heart disease and cancer than did those who didn't take the pills. Another study from the National Cancer Institute reported that men who took vitamin E were much more likely to develop prostate cancer. While that news is a little disturbing, it probably just means that these people were already in poor health when they sought out the supplements, suggests David Katz, MD, nutrition expert at Yale School of Medicine.

In other words, there's no indication that the increased risks seen in these studies were caused by the pills, Dr. Katz says. Often people who take multivitamins do so because they're already sick, or at risk for a disease—which could account for the differences in longevity between pill-takers and avoiders. "However," he says, "by isolating the vitamins and minerals in these foods, we may be getting the dose wrong, or perhaps the nutrients need other ingredients—present in the food but not the pill—to work."

Be Careful Not to Overdo It

Consider vitamin B9: Also known as folate (or, in synthetic form, as folic acid), the vitamin plays a role in heart health and nerve development; it's also a basic building block in the formation of new cells. Since 1996, the Food and Drug Administration has required that all grains be fortified with folic acid because it helps pregnant women get enough of this B vitamin to protect their fetuses from neural tube defects.

All well and good—but that means the folic acid in multivitamins is superfluous. Even worse, it could raise the risk of breast cancer in women. Swedish researchers looked at data on more than 35,000 women and found that multivitamin takers were 19% more likely to develop breast cancer. Of course, in a study of this size it's tough to control for all the potential nutrients in the women's diet— and lifestyle behaviors—that could have contributed to the increased risk.

As Katz points out, there's no need to panic if you take supplements. And some nutrients make a lot of sense to get from a pill, such as omega-3 fats for people who don't like fish and vitamin D for people who live in areas where the winter is long and the sun is scarce. But if you have a healthy lifestyle, you may want to think twice before you commit to taking multivitamins.

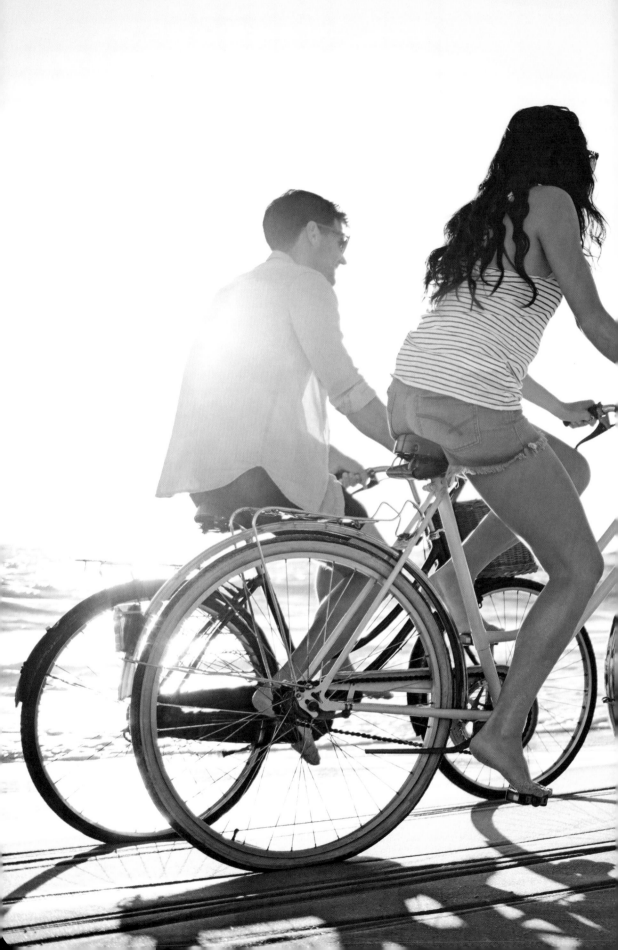

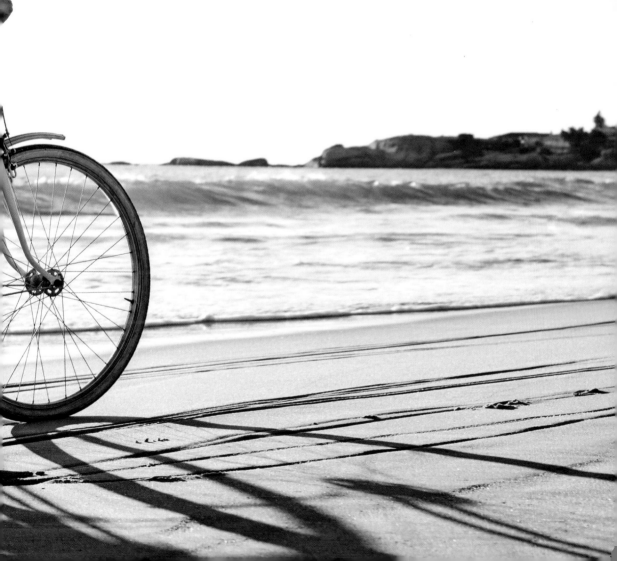

Chapter 2

THE POWER OF SUPPLEMENTS

FEEL YOUNGER, LOSE WEIGHT, GET ENERGY,
IMPROVE LIBIDO AND BOLSTER YOUR IMMUNITY.

HAVING MORE ENERGY IS EASY WITH THE RIGHT STUFF.

Much of what we consider to be normal aging is actually just symptoms of mild malnutrition.

Stay Young

THE FOUNTAIN OF YOUTH MAY BE DOWN AT
YOUR DRUGSTORE—SO LONG AS YOU CHOOSE WISELY.

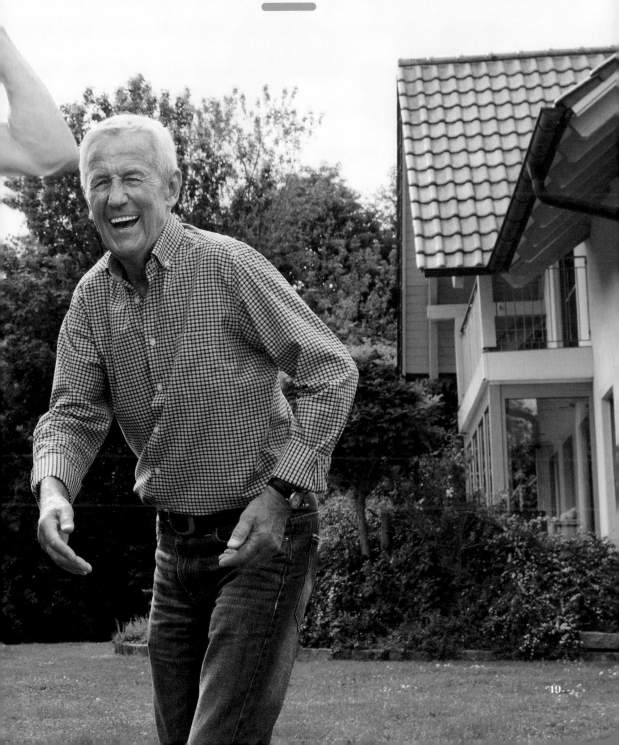

A h, youth: Actually, no one wants to revisit the folly of their younger years. But to have the skin, the health, the vigor? Yes, please. Unfortunately, many anti-aging products offer more wild claims than actual improvements. But the following supplements at least have some evidence that they can keep Father Time at bay just a little bit longer.

Turn Back the Clock

Arginine is an amino acid with a reputation for stimulating your pituitary gland, which is responsible for growth hormone—the stuff that keeps your metabolism humming and your muscles supple. It also improves your blood circulation, and that can have a positive effect on your sex life. A common dosage to start with is 2 grams daily.

Live Longer

The herb astragalus has so many tricks up its sleeve. One of the most intriguing secrets is that in some research, astragalus has been shown to elongate telomeres, the fragile ends of your DNA that grow shorter as you get older as part of the normal aging process. Longer telomeres are associated with improved longevity, cardiovascular health, cognition and immune functioning. Take 25 to 50 mg of this herb daily. Look for astragalosides, compounds extracted from the astragalus herb.

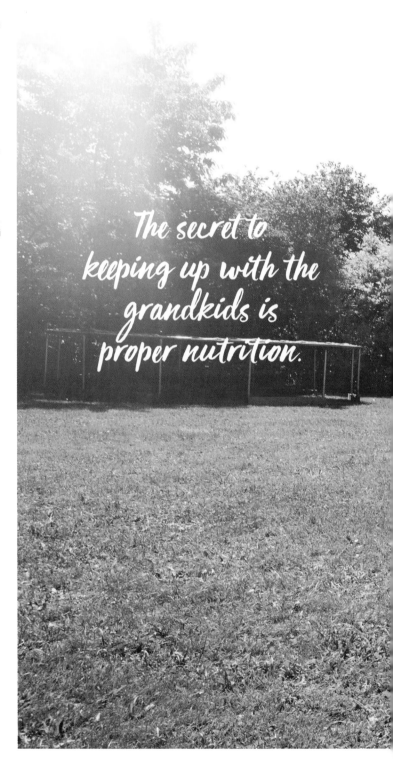

The secret to keeping up with the grandkids is proper nutrition.

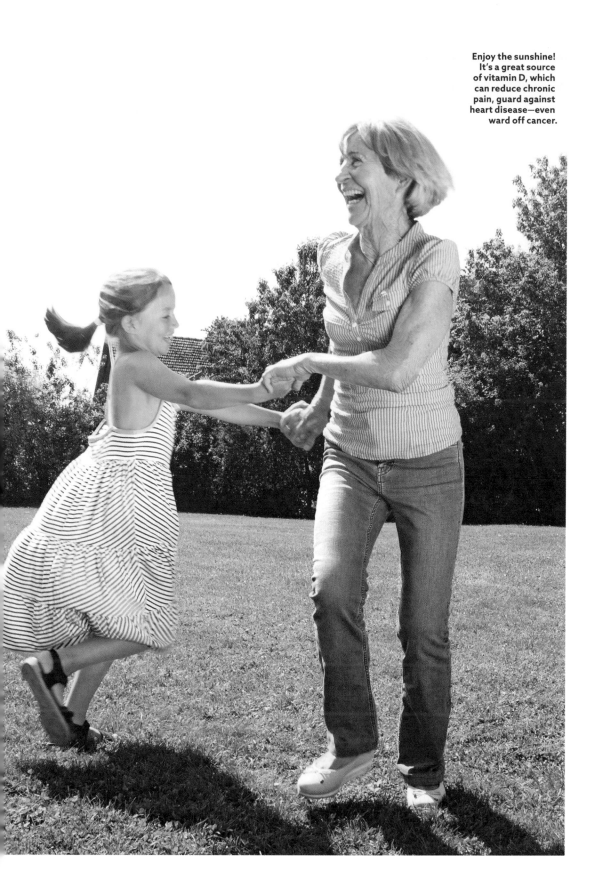

Enjoy the sunshine! It's a great source of vitamin D, which can reduce chronic pain, guard against heart disease—even ward off cancer.

→ **You might benefit from a supplement, but don't overdo it. Megadoses can be dangerous.**

Get Healthy, Glowing Skin

This one is a mouthful: polypodium leucotomos extract. You can just call it PLE—and if you're concerned about aging skin, you might be interested in this supplement. Taken from a tropical fern, PLE has been tested in published research. A study in the *Journal of Photochemistry and Photobiology* suggests the extract can help preserve the supportive architecture of your skin, called fibroblasts. By building and restoring collagen, it helps prevent—and potentially alleviate—wrinkles and sagging skin. It could even play a role in preventing sun damage, according to research published in the *International Journal of Dermatology*. By making the skin more resistant to UV damage, PLE allows your skin to withstand more sun exposure—and it could reduce the risk of skin cancer. In studies, people typically take about 500 mg a day.

Because the sun is so hard on your skin, you should also make sure you're getting selenium— it seems to help protect against skin aging and skin cancers. It

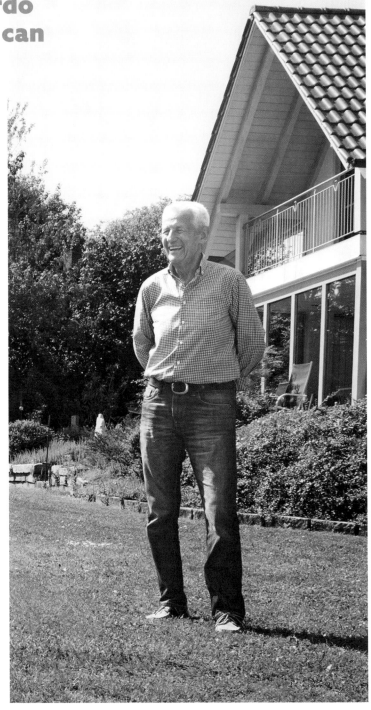

supports collagen and can help maintain skin elasticity. Some good food sources of the mineral include seafood, garlic, whole grains and eggs.

Animal research on the mineral appears even more promising: Studies suggest that when researchers gave animals L-selenomethionine —a form of selenium—it helped ward off skin cancer.

Keep Your Heart and Brain Fit

Resveratrol is a polyphenol—a group of compounds that have antioxidant abilities: They prevent the kind of cell damage that can lead to cancer, for example. Research suggests it can reduce inflammation, which can help battle heart disease; it also lowers LDL ("bad") cholesterol and helps thin the blood, reducing the risk

of clots that can lead to heart attacks. It also seems to slow the buildup of the type of brain plaque that researchers have linked to Alzheimer's disease.

You can get resveratrol from eating grapes or by drinking red wine in moderation. (White wine doesn't contain as much because resveratrol is in the skins, and the skins are removed earlier in the fermentation process.) But you can also get the nutrient from peanuts, blueberries and cranberries. Most supplements deliver about 250 to 500 mg of the compound.

Protect Your Mind and Your Face

Chocolate contains antioxidants known as cocoa flavanols that may offer a big boost for your brain and your heart. A study published in the journal *Nature Neuroscience* suggests that flavanols can act directly on the brain to reduce age-related cognitive decline. Regular cocoa flavanol consumption also has positive effects on facial wrinkles

and elasticity, according to a study from the *Journal of Nutrition*. Research suggests you need more than you can get in a bar of dark chocolate, so try a daily supplement with 1,000 mg.

Pollution Blocker

Vitamin C is the most common antioxidant found in the skin, which means it's also the one you tend to lose fastest if your skin is frequently exposed to airborne pollution and the ultraviolet rays in sunlight. As your body's C levels start to diminish, your skin will begin to sustain more and more damage from environmental stressors. Some research suggests that a combination of sun and pollution can deplete your C stores by as much as 55%. Try supplementing with 100 mg or more (up to 1,000 mg) daily.

WATCH OUT FOR SNAKE OIL

Buying skin creams stocked with exotic vitamins may only empty your wallet faster, say the experts at the American Academy of Dermatology. Although the active ingredients—namely, antioxidants—can prevent skin damage by blocking dangerous free radicals, the reality is your skin absorbs little from the products. Most of your benefit comes from the moisturizing effects of the creams.

Be wary of too-good-to-be-true claims as well. The FDA recently forced the company Strivectin to alter language on a cream that asserted: "Clinically proven to change the anatomy of a wrinkle." Why? The FDA says that's a drug-like effect, and the company would have to get approval to sell something so powerful. However, the American Chemical Society points out there's just not enough of the good stuff in the products to have a drug-like effect. Do yourself a favor—and save money—by avoiding products that make outrageous promises.

You can jump-start your weight loss with certain nutrients.

THESE INGREDIENTS MAY PROVIDE THE EXTRA PUSH YOU NEED.

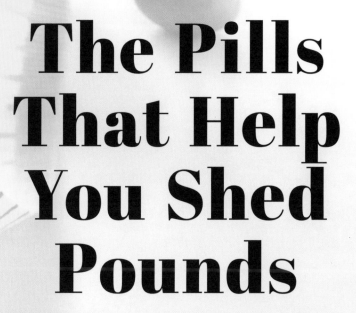

The Pills That Help You Shed Pounds

LOSING WEIGHT IS TOUGH—YOU CAN USE ALL THE SUPPORT YOU CAN GET.

Y ou know that to really slim down, your best bet is a smart diet that controls or reduces calories, not to mention plenty of exercise. But we all know how tough it is to lose weight. Remember *The Biggest Loser*? When researchers at the National Institutes of Health tracked contestants who had lost more than 125 pounds over six years, all but one had regained the weight, even though they continued to diet and exercise.

Clearly, dieters can use all the help they can find. While there is no magic pill that will make you effortlessly drop dozens of pounds, there are some supplements that may assist your efforts. Just make sure that you continue to eat properly and drink plenty of water; it's easy to get dehydrated when you're trying to lose weight. As always, check with your doctor to make sure the pills don't interfere with any medications you might be taking or worsen any conditions—diabetes, heart disease—that you may have.

Chitosan

Made from the shells of lobsters, crabs and shrimp, this sugar seems to interfere with the absorption of calories. The evidence for chitosan is a bit mixed at the moment, but one large analysis of research that was published in the *Journal of Obesity* suggests that when people took this supplement with food, they dropped body fat and struggled less with bloating. In most research, people have taken 1,500 mg, twice a day, with meals.

The substance behaves like fiber when it hits the digestive tract: In animal studies, scientists have found that chitosan binds with fat and ushers it through the intestines before it can be digested. When chitosan is coupled with regular workouts, the supplement tends to be more helpful. Researchers at Loyola University Medical Center in Maywood, Illinois, put 30 overweight patients on an exercise program and gave them either 2,000 mg a day of chitosan or a placebo. After four months, the chitosan group lost an average of 15 pounds, compared to the placebo group's

6 pounds. Chitosan also lowered bad cholesterol nearly four times as much, compared to the placebo, and it almost doubled levels of good cholesterol.

Should you decide to try it, remember: It comes from shellfish, so it can trigger a reaction in people who are allergic to shellfish. And because chitosan also binds with fluids, you'll need to take it with plenty of water—at least 8 ounces with each pill.

Conjugated Linoleic Acid (CLA)

This healthy fat found in meat and dairy helps burn fat and build muscle. CLA isn't magic; people taking the highest effective dose—3.2 grams a day—typically lose close to a pound of body fat per month (in addition to whatever they're losing through other weight-loss efforts). Because it also boosts muscle, the overall drop in pounds isn't that impressive—but the health advantage is. Fat buildup is linked to chronic conditions such as heart disease and diabetes, while extra muscle is associated with a faster metabolism and longevity.

The best food sources of CLA tend to be grass-fed beef, organic milk, cheese, yogurt and eggs. Most weight-loss regimens can accommodate an egg a day, three to four servings of lean beef each week and two to three daily servings of dairy—or you can find supplements at most drugstores.

Green Coffee Beans

Coffee has long been given credit for a number of health benefits, including weight loss when taken in moderation, along with improved glycemic response to

reduce diabetes risk. And while caffeine itself may play a role (it has a thermogenic effect, which can stimulate metabolism and spur slight weight loss), there are also other substances in the beans themselves which may hold some promise when it comes to fighting obesity. One of these is chlorogenic acid, a dietary phenol found in green coffee beans that is extracted before roasting. (The roasting process breaks down some of the beans' biologically active properties.)

A 2011 British meta-analysis looked at the effectiveness of green coffee bean extract in human clinical trials and found a modest decrease (about 5 pounds) in body weight for those who received green coffee bean extract compared with a placebo. Researchers caution, however, that sample sizes were limited and no long-term effects were tracked.

A small study out of Korea found similar results in a group of 23 overweight women, who had modest reduction of body weight after taking a green coffee bean extract over an eight-week period compared to those who took a placebo. The subjects also had a slight decrease in body fat percentage, including total fat and visceral (abdominal) fat.

Green coffee bean extract is sold as a pill; a typical dose is between 60 and 185 mg a day.

Green Tea

The grassy flavor of green tea may put you off, but you may not have to develop a taste for it to reap the benefits. Green tea contains plant compounds called catechins, including epigallocatechin-3-gallate (EGCG). Catechins, also found in black tea and oolong in

WHAT ABOUT RX WEIGHT-LOSS PILLS?

Given the obesity issue in the United States, it's no surprise pharmaceutical companies are trying to develop medications that can help melt pounds. Their success has been less than stellar: The weight loss is minimal, although some people find the drugs helpful. One note is that most of the drugs are approved only for people who are obese (they have a body mass index [BMI] of 30 or higher; if you're 5 feet, 6 inches tall, for example, you'd have to weigh more than 185 pounds) or for people who have a BMI of 27 along with a weight-related condition such as diabetes or high blood pressure. Here are some options.

》 ALLI/XENICAL
(ORLISTAT)
What to Expect
This chemical actually helps block the absorption of fat, and it can bring about a 10% to 15% loss in people who respond well. But as is true with many of these prescriptions, not everyone experiences these results.

Side Effects
These drugs can cause loose stools and prevent nutrient absorption, so avoid high-fat meals (which can cause digestive distress) and take a multivitamin.

》 CONTRAVE
(NALTREXONE/BUPROPION)
What to Expect
This combo targets the brain's center for appetite and metabolism. It came about because as separate drugs, each led to weight loss—about 13.5% of total weight.
Side Effects
Nausea, headache, vomiting, diarrhea, trouble sleeping

》 QSYMIA
(PHENTERMINE/TOPIRAMATE)
What to Expect
By boosting the appetite-regulating hormone leptin, this often produces good results. Users can drop about 20 pounds, on average, after a year on the pill—with some people losing even more.
Side Effects
People with eye problems, such as glaucoma, or who have experienced suicidal thoughts should not take this drug.

》 SAXENDA
(LIRAGLUTIDE)
What to Expect
Given as an injection, it mimics an intestinal hormone that helps stifle appetite. Over a year, volunteers lost an average of 18 pounds.
Side Effects
Vomiting, severe diarrhea or constipation; some users experience low blood sugar.

》 WEGOVY
(SEMAGLUTIDE)
What to Expect
Newly approved for weight loss, this drug got its start as a treatment for type 2 diabetes in a lower dosage, and works to suppress appetite in the brain. In trials, nearly a third of subjects lost up to 20% of their body weight on the medication.
Side Effects
Although experts say it's well tolerated, side effects can include nausea, diarrhea, vomiting, constipation and stomach pain.

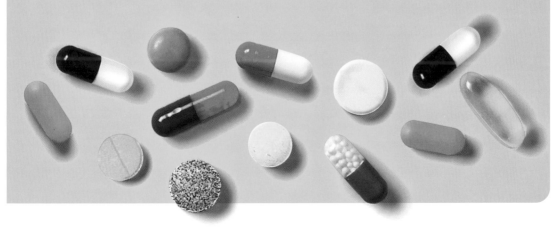

lesser amounts, seem to protect natural stimulants in the body. More of this stimulant equals higher cell activity throughout your body, increasing your need for energy. Suddenly you're burning more calories just sitting around.

Your weight loss will vary with catechins; just don't expect too much. Researchers at the Cleveland Clinic analyzed the results of 15 studies on catechin supplements and found that pills could help you lose about a pound a month. The catechins seemed to stimulate the body to burn more fat, resulting in significantly narrower waists among supplement takers. That finding ties in with long-term observational studies: Green tea drinkers who have about two cups a day have a lower percentage of body fat and thinner waists than nondrinkers do.

Experts believe green tea may be most useful to dieters hoping to prevent weight regain. Dieting depresses metabolism, and green tea can help counteract that drop. If you want to try supplements, the effective dose seems to be about 600 mg a day. Be sure to get pills with caffeine: The Cleveland Clinic study indicated that caffeine-free supplements don't help.

Pyruvate

This relatively unknown supplement is actually produced by your body as a by-product of sugar digestion. The compound has been synthesized—and when given to overweight people, it seems to encourage fat-burning in the body. In a study of 51 men and women who took 6 grams a day, combined with a healthy diet and regular exercise, pyruvate led to body-fat losses of 12%, on average. However, people who struggle with irritable bowel syndrome may want to avoid the supplement—it can make symptoms worse.

Whey Protein

You know that watery stuff on the top of your yogurt? Don't scoop it off: It's whey protein, and it can help you shed weight. In numerous studies, dieters who tried whey supplements or shakes lost only a bit more weight than those using other types of protein supplements, but they did gain one distinct advantage: Whey dieters shed about twice as much body fat as nonwhey dieters (who tend to lose a combination of fat, muscle and other lean tissue).

The best sources of whey include ricotta cheese, goat cheese, milk, cottage cheese and regular yogurt. Whey protein can also be found in many energy bars and protein shakes. Just don't overdo it: Roughly 20 grams a day is plenty for people getting regular exercise. If you're adding whey protein supplements to your diet, consider taking about 1 to 2 grams a day.

TAKE NOTE

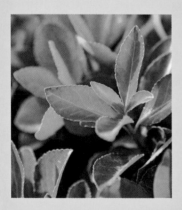

If you're not a big tea drinker, you can still get the active ingredients of green tea in pill form.

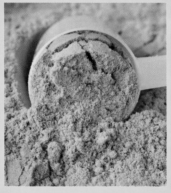

A 2008 study revealed that dieters who drank whey-protein shakes as meal replacements lost fat and not muscle.

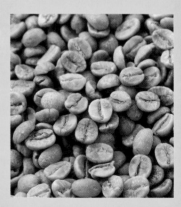

Grind up unroasted coffee beans, and you might find that you get a diet-saving boost from the powder.

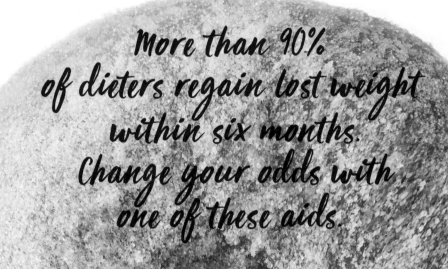

More than 90%
of dieters regain lost weight
within six months.
Change your odds with
one of these aids.

Even if you have quite
a bit to lose, set reasonable
goals. Remember: Studies
indicate that losing
just 5% of your body
weight means better
cholesterol, lower blood
pressure and a longer life.

Fight Fatigue & Get Your Energy Back

WITH THE RIGHT SUPPLEMENTS, YOU CAN FEEL YOUR BEST EVERY DAY.

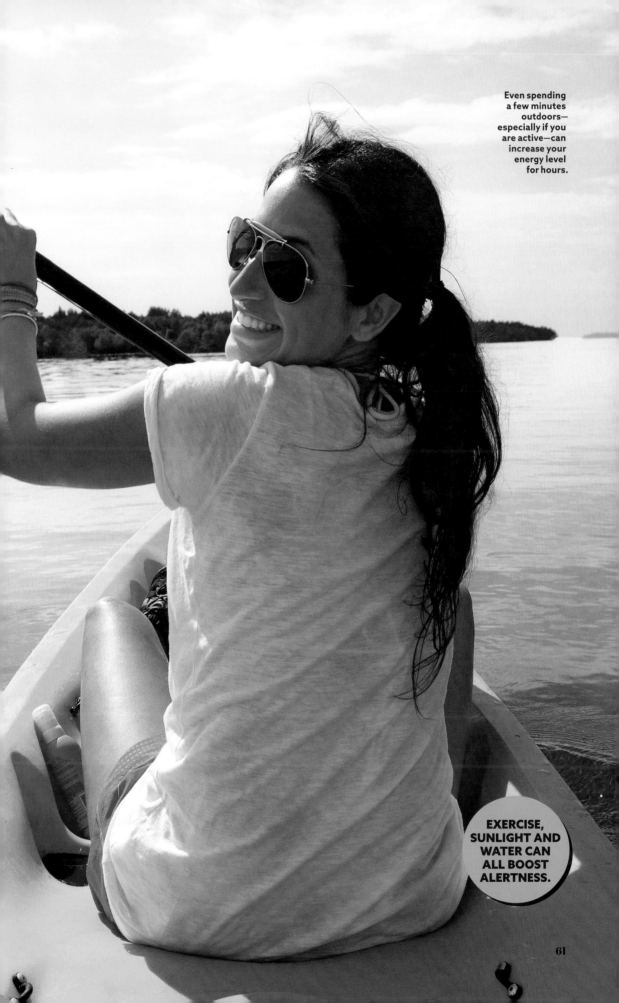

Even spending a few minutes outdoors—especially if you are active—can increase your energy level for hours.

EXERCISE, SUNLIGHT AND WATER CAN ALL BOOST ALERTNESS.

L ife is a lot tougher when you're tapped out. Whether it's because you're sleeping poorly, or stress is sapping your reserves, you have to find a way to turn fatigue around. Paul Baard, PhD, a sports psychologist at Fordham University in New York, points out that running on empty robs you of strength and willpower, allowing bad habits to take over: You don't exercise, you make bad food choices and your energy dips even lower.

Reverse the cycle with targeted supplementation. You can avoid the lulls, lags and dips in your vitality with the options below. Learn how to keep your tank full and your engine racing.

Ashwagandha

If anxiety is draining your energy, this may be the herb for you. Promising research on ashwagandha suggests that it could be helpful for protecting against Alzheimer's disease, but that's just one of its tricks—and the reason the herb is known as an adaptogen in traditional forms of medicine. Research has found that ashwagandha can relieve insomnia and stress-induced depression—two conditions that can rob you of energy. And in a three-month study of 87 people suffering from anxiety and depression, ashwagandha supplements—300 mg, twice a day—relieved symptoms dramatically while boosting energy, compared to volunteers taking a placebo. While researchers are still testing the herb to learn more, experts suggests that taking 500 mg of

→ **Stress is a big contributor to fatigue, so do your best to minimize your obligations.**

ashwagandha a day could help tame worry, boost your mood and increase your energy.

Cocoa

This qualifies as the best health news in decades: Chocolate is really, really good for you. The fat in chocolate—cocoa butter—is equal parts monounsaturated (the healthy kind of fat) and a relatively benign type of saturated fat called stearic acid. Unlike most saturated fats, stearic acid doesn't seem to raise cholesterol, and it may even help lower bad cholesterol.

Cocoa—or cacao—also contains flavonoids—antioxidants typically found in produce that help protect against heart disease. Research suggests that eating small amounts of chocolate can increase the amount of nitric oxide—a substance that helps keep blood vessels relaxed and pumping smoothly—in the bloodstream. That's not only great for your heart and for keeping blood pressure down, but it means that you're getting a steady flow of oxygen and nutrients to your muscles and organs. And that will lead to an increase in energy levels; when people with mild to moderate fatigue got cocoa flavanols, they reported feeling much better.

The best way to get chocolate is by eating it, of course. The only hitch is that you have to eat dark chocolate—at least 60% cocoa

(the packaging will indicate the percentage). Milk chocolate is only about 25% cocoa, so it won't make much of an antioxidant impact. An ounce or two of dark chocolate—a couple of squares from the typical bar—daily is plenty. Not a fan of dark chocolate? Try a daily 500 mg cocoa-extract supplement.

Coenzyme Q10

This enzyme, often abbreviated as CoQ10, helps the machinery in cells convert carbohydrates into a type of energy known as adenosine triphosphate—the gasoline that powers your body. That makes it central to energy production; clearly, getting enough can help give you a boost. When researchers have given it to people with chronic fatigue or fibromyalgia, the patients reported feeling much better. It also increased vitality in the elderly in one study. That's significant, because we tend to produce less of this vital substance as we age.

CoQ10 can also help cells dispose of cell waste, which aids in workout recovery. In a study from Iran, researchers found that giving the enzyme to runners before a workout led to much quicker and easier recoveries: The runners who got CoQ10 had less inflammation and reported less fatigue than a group who got a placebo.

What's more, the enzyme has antioxidant properties that prevent fats such as cholesterol and triglycerides from damaging your arteries. That's a lot of pluses for one nutrient! Since CoQ10 levels decline with age, it's important to make sure that you get some from food sources, to assist in correcting any mild deficiencies. And you may just find you have more energy for those calorie-blasting workouts.

This compound is found in fish, red meat, eggs and, to a lesser degree, in spinach, broccoli and nuts. As a supplement, you can get it in two forms: ubiquinol and ubiquinone. Because nearly 90% of the CoQ10 in your blood is ubiquinol, it makes sense to look for this version of the supplement. People take between 90 and 200 mg per day.

Cordyceps

This fungus happens to grow in certain caterpillars in the Himalayas. How anyone ever figured out that it could battle fatigue is lost to history, but you'll be relieved to hear that scientists have been able to successfully grow cordyceps in a lab, bringing the cost way down.

In research, cordyceps appears to facilitate oxygen uptake, increasing your endurance. Other findings suggest it can also stimulate the immune system, helping you ward off the type of low-level illnesses that can drain energy. According to Andrew Weil, MD, cordyceps is used to combat fatigue and lift your mental energy and mood. Because it seems to assist in controlling blood sugar, cordyceps may at some point prove helpful against diabetes; smoothing the highs and lows

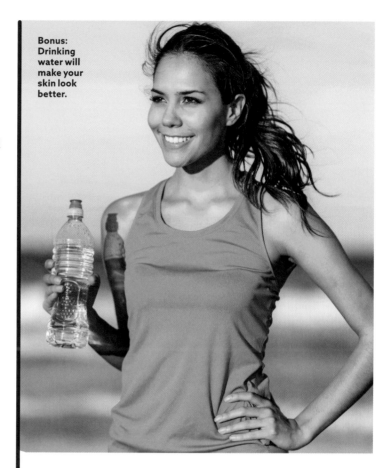

Bonus: Drinking water will make your skin look better.

ALL NATURAL

Energy Boosters

Water//
Every cell in your body depends on fluids to function properly. You can even boost your outlook and energy. Researchers have found that mild dehydration, which starts when you fall to 98.5% of your body's 100% water volume, can muddy thinking and reaction times, leaving you fatigued. To avoid a slump, aim to drink 10–15 cups of water throughout the day.

Exercise//
It may sound counterintuitive when you're tired, but even small amounts of physical activity can increase energy. Just getting up and taking a walk will help circulate more oxygen throughout the body.

of blood sugar can also even out mood and prevent energy dips. Follow the advice on the label, since amounts can vary.

Ginseng

Like ashwagandha, ginseng is an adaptogen thought to treat a variety of troubles by boosting the immune system and easing stress. It comes in several types; the most common are American and Panax (or Asian) ginseng.

American ginseng seems to offer the clearest energy-boosting benefits, although Panax ginseng may help relieve anxiety and depression. Researchers have found that 400 mg a day of Panax could help calm study volunteers, improve their ability to solve problems and ease stress.

In studies of American ginseng, cancer patients who were battling fatigue took 1,000 mg of the supplement twice a day for two months and reportedly improved energy levels by 51%. That's a big dose, so discuss it with your doctor before you start supplementing. It's also important to realize that the people in the cancer study were very sick; for people with average energy depletion, a dose of 100 to 400 mg a day could be plenty.

Siberian ginseng—also called eleuthero—is completely different from the other ginsengs. There's some evidence it may help relieve chronic fatigue. A study involving 96 patients revealed that after a couple of months, the patients had far more energy than did a group taking a placebo.

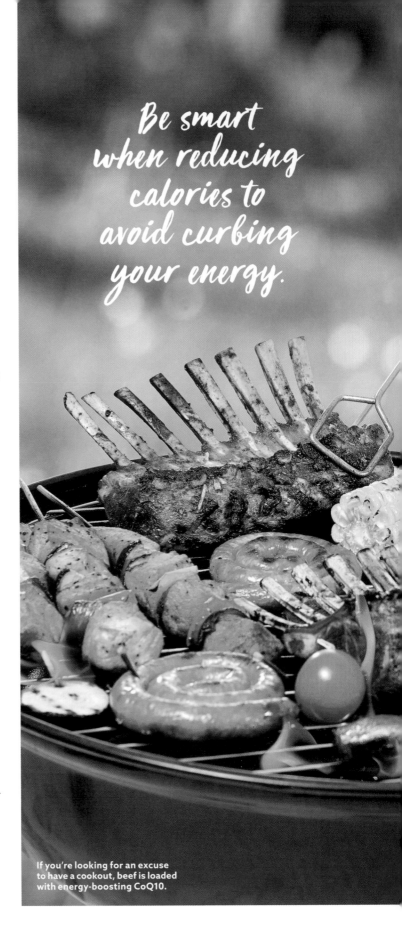

Be smart when reducing calories to avoid curbing your energy.

If you're looking for an excuse to have a cookout, beef is loaded with energy-boosting CoQ10.

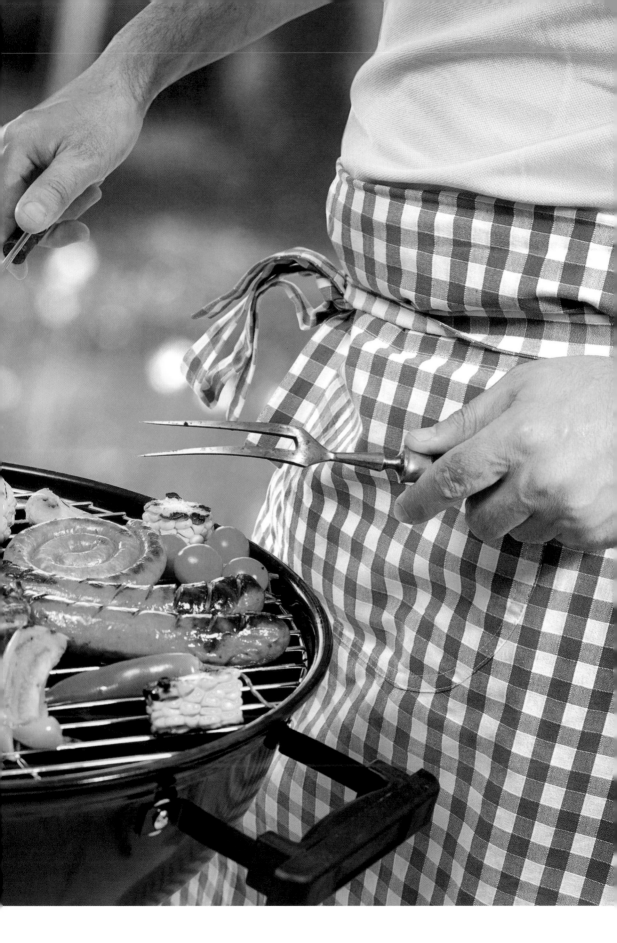

Libido Boosters

SPICE THINGS UP WITHOUT PHARMACEUTICALS.

ARGININE

Your body converts this amino acid into nitric oxide, which dilates and relaxes blood vessels. Combined with another herb called yohimbe, it can help treat erectile dysfunction—but use caution, since the substances can trigger stomach upset, increased heart rate and other side effects. Some research suggests taking between 2 and 5 grams a day.

GINSENG

Canadian researchers have found that ginseng can help men struggling with erectile dysfunction. It seems to boost energy and raise testosterone, enhancing sexual responsiveness in both men and women. Some research suggests 3 grams of Korean red ginseng daily.

FENUGREEK

This clover-like plant is found in the Mediterranean and Western Asia, and researchers have found that in supplement form it can slow the absorption of sugar and stimulate insulin, helping control blood sugar. It also seems to encourage libido: In two different studies published in *Phytotherapy Research*, results suggest that men and women who took 600 mg a day for six weeks reported increases in sexual arousal, energy and stamina. Women may benefit from the herb's ability to ease the symptoms of painful menstruation, as well.

GINKGO

Substances in the leaves and seeds of this ancient tree can be made into teas and pills that encourage blood flow and relax muscles. And unlike many supposed aphrodisiacs, women seem to benefit from gingko's effects as well as men; in combination with sex therapy, the herb proved to be useful in raising women's libido. Experts recommend starting with no more than 120 mg a day.

MACA ROOT

This high-elevation Andes plant has been popular for boosting energy and increasing immunity. Ground-up maca root has also been used as a way to treat anemia and fight off illness. And it's been touted as a pick-me-up in the bedroom for both men and women, for a number of conditions —as well as a general aphrodisiac. A study published in the journal *Evidence-Based Complementary and Alternative Medicine* suggests that it helps balance male and female sex hormones as well as boost fertility. While you can find maca teas and drinks, the most common way to get it is in powdered capsules. Most research suggests a dose between 1.5 and 3 grams a day.

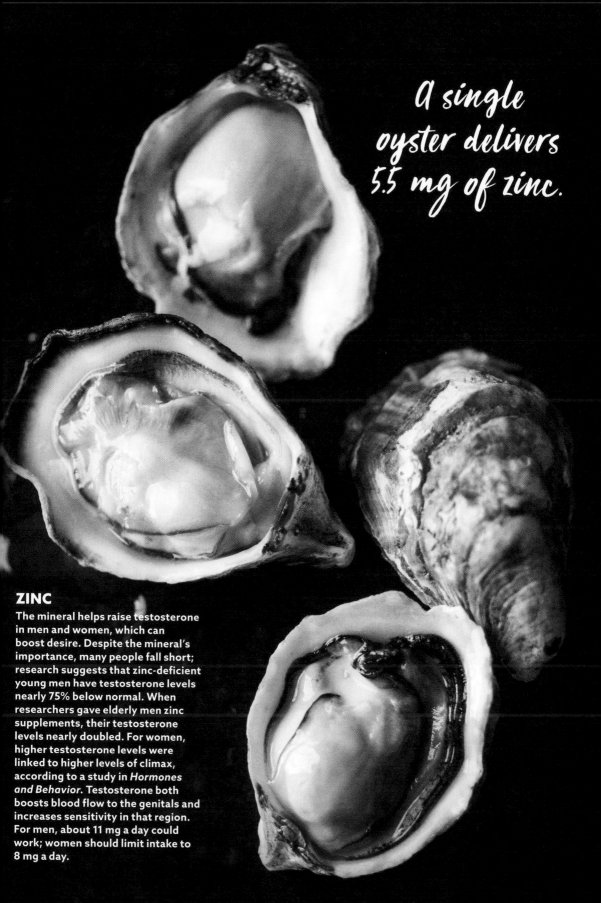

A single oyster delivers 5.5 mg of zinc.

ZINC

The mineral helps raise testosterone in men and women, which can boost desire. Despite the mineral's importance, many people fall short; research suggests that zinc-deficient young men have testosterone levels nearly 75% below normal. When researchers gave elderly men zinc supplements, their testosterone levels nearly doubled. For women, higher testosterone levels were linked to higher levels of climax, according to a study in *Hormones and Behavior*. Testosterone both boosts blood flow to the genitals and increases sensitivity in that region. For men, about 11 mg a day could work; women should limit intake to 8 mg a day.

FIRE UP YOUR BRAIN CELLS WITH NATURAL AIDS.

Smart Ways to Stay Sharp

GET AN EDGE, WITH SUBSTANCES THAT KEEP YOUR NEURONS FIRING.

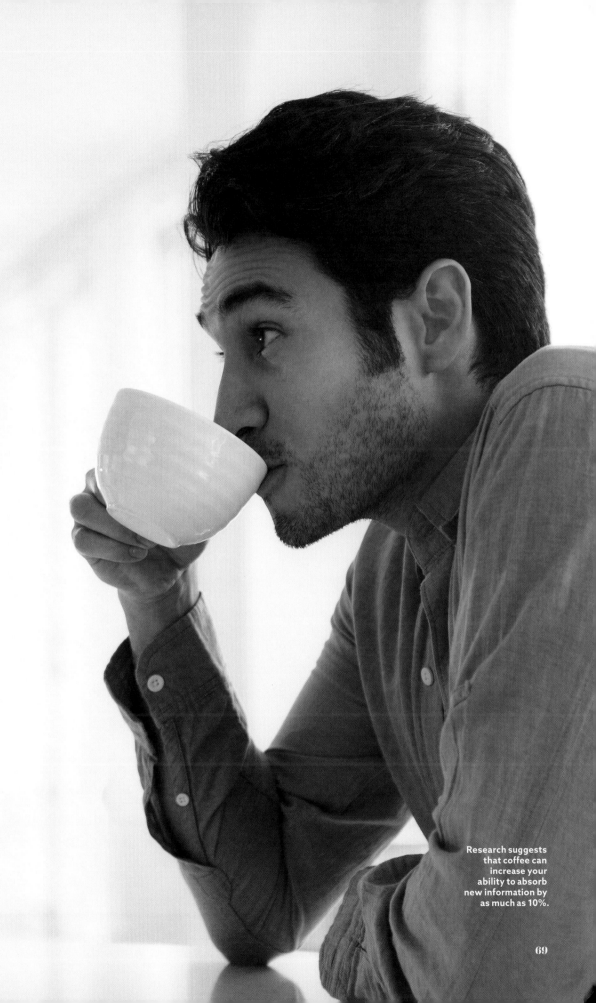

Research suggests that coffee can increase your ability to absorb new information by as much as 10%.

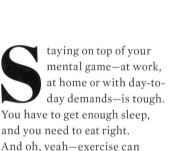

Build a High-Performance Mind

Drink Coffee

Would you believe that coffee is one of the top sources of antioxidants in the American diet? It's true, although the reason for that probably has more to do with the average American's failure to eat enough produce.

Still, it's time to revise java's bad reputation: Your morning cup of joe is a rich source of several healthy substances—particularly of a phenol called chlorogenic acid. It can help your body manage blood sugar while boosting circulation—two things that benefit your brain.

Even better, the combination of chlorogenic acid and caffeine appears to increase short-term recall; in several studies that tested the cognitive function of adults, coffee drinkers had faster reaction times, better verbal memory and improved reasoning. If you don't like coffee or caffeinated tea, you could try supplements. You can also get the good stuff from coffee in green coffee bean extract: Start at around 120 mg and remember to take the supplements early in the day (as you would coffee) or you'll risk interrupting your sleep.

Savor Sage

It's a great seasoning for potatoes or chicken, but sage pills could help your mind: People who took doses of common sage or Spanish sage have performed better on tests of memory and focus in several studies. Even smelling this herb can help. In one study, researchers gave healthy volunteers (aged 18 to 37) sage oil and then tested their word recall over the following several hours. People getting sage outperformed those who got a placebo by up to 10%. Sage seems to slow the breakdown of crucial neurotransmitters. In studies, subjects have typically taken around 1 gram a day of sage oil.

Get Some Ginseng

When you want better focus, this herb may be the answer. It's been a popular brain-boosting supplement for a long time, with a reputation for helping out in moments of high intellectual demand: When researchers gave volunteers Panax ginseng, they discovered that the herb could boost scores on tests of problem-solving and focus. Children with ADHD who get the herb have much better attention to detail and fewer symptoms of hyperactivity. The typical dose is 200 to 400 mg, twice daily.

Try Tyrosine

Prepping for a big presentation? This amino acid could be exactly what you need. When taken by people under the stress of heavy work demands, tyrosine helps improve mental performance and memory. Volunteers who were

Staying on top of your mental game—at work, at home or with day-to-day demands—is tough. You have to get enough sleep, and you need to eat right. And oh, yeah—exercise can do wonders for your mind. But what happens when the responsibilities pile up, sleep is elusive and you don't really have time to keep up with a complete diet?

That's where the right nutrients can help you keep your wits about you. First, you need a sane approach. When you think about it, there are three important aspects to your mind to target: 1) You want a high-performing brain that really shines in big meetings and when you're up against big deadlines; 2) You need a memory that's capable of accurate, lightning-fast recall; and 3) You must do your best to remain brain-healthy as you age, so you can ward off dementia. After all, why can't you be one of those centenarians who is sharp as a tack? You may be, if you make the effort to approach your supplement strategy with care. Take on each of these challenges with the following nutrients and be ready to wow your co-workers, family members and friends.

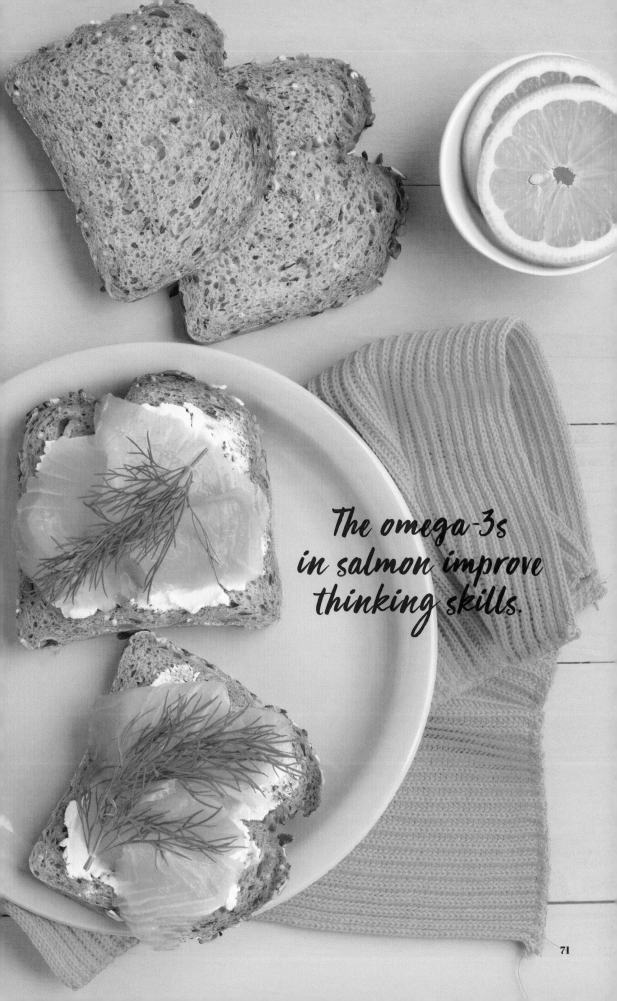

The omega-3s
in salmon improve
thinking skills.

sleep-deprived, undergoing boot camp–style training or subjected to loud, distracting noises performed much better on tests of decision-making, problem-solving and recall when taking tyrosine. The usual dose is around 150 mg per kilogram of body weight. (A kilogram is 2.2 pounds.)

Make More of Your Memory

Find Some Fish Oil

If you're not eating fish on a regular basis, you're depriving your memory. Fish oil is a rich source of docosahexaenoic acid (DHA) and eicosapentaenoic acid (EPA), two types of healthy omega-3 fatty acids, and your brain depends on these fats: DHA accounts for about 25% of the total fat in brain cells.

Some research suggests that supplements improve your recall, not to mention your thinking skills and reaction times. In a study of 18- to 25-year-olds taking fish-oil supplements, researchers found that the pills could boost memory performance by 23%. The speculation is that the effect may be even greater for people in middle age or older. While some of the evidence that DHA and EPA could protect against natural aging of the brain hasn't held up, the research on omega-3s and memory seems to be getting stronger. A great way to get these healthy omega-3 fats is to get two servings of oily fish—think salmon, mackerel, sardines or anchovies—per week. If fish isn't your favorite, aim for a gram's worth of supplements per day.

Boost Blood Flow

To deliver the nutrients and fats your brain requires, your circulation must be strong. This helps explain why acetyl-L-carnitine—an amino acid—can help your recall. Researchers have found that taking supplements of acetyl-L-carnitine improves short-term memory. In another study, researchers gave it to mice under stress and found that it could prevent damage to the amygdala, a structure in the brain that controls emotions and memory. In fact, research indicates that people over the age of 30 seem to recall

→ **One in five people will suffer from some form of dementia. Take action before it's too late.**

information better when they take acetyl-L-carnitine. In most studies, the daily target has been around 1,500 mg, split into two to three doses.

Keep Decay at Bay

You Can't Beat Bacopa

Bacopa monnieri is a medicine made from the herb of the same name. It's popular in traditional herbal medicine such as Ayurveda.

Commonly prescribed by natural healers for brain function, bacopa monnieri has been found to improve thinking skills and memory in people

who are experiencing a decline, as well as those who are completely healthy. Researchers have typically studied a dosage of about 300 mg a day; one thing to note is that you have to take it regularly to notice a benefit. In studies, volunteers typically take it for four to six weeks to gain benefits. Take it with food, by the way: Some research suggests it can cause an upset stomach.

Best Get Some B Vitamins

Specifically: folate, vitamin B12 and vitamin B6 (pyridoxine). According to Michael Greger, MD, of nutritionfacts.org, your body needs the vitamins to manage levels of an amino acid called homocysteine.

Many are familiar with the way homocysteine can harm the heart. Dr. Greger is concerned with what it can do to the brain: People with genetic mutations that lead to high levels of the amino acid suffer brain damage; even slightly elevated levels can increase the risk of Alzheimer's disease. Getting enough of these B vitamins seems to tame homocysteine and preserve brain volume (brain atrophy is a key part of dementia). You can get them from a well-rounded diet—or consider a B-complex supplement.

TRAINING YOUR BRAIN

You go to the gym for your body; why should your brain get short shrift? If you want to keep your mind fit, take these steps.

STAY SOCIAL

Say yes to parties, trivia nights, coffee with friends—and while you're at it, sign up for some extended-learning classes. Keeping your brain active through learning and socializing may help delay or ward off dementia, according to brain experts. In one study, 92% of elderly people who were assigned to take college-level courses showed impressive increases in their ability to think and reason, compared to a control group. And research from the National Institutes of Health found that training the brain through specific exercises could offer mental-processing benefits for a decade or more.

PLAY GAMES

The research on whether doing the daily crossword or playing sudoku benefits your brain is contradictory. However, memory researchers still believe that the mental stimulation of playing games makes a difference in how well your brain ages. So by all means, play chess, backgammon or bridge, do crosswords, and keep reading books, whether fiction or nonfiction. Just be sure to mix up the challenge for the most benefit. By continually surprising and making new demands on your mind, you can ensure that your brain will form new neural connections.

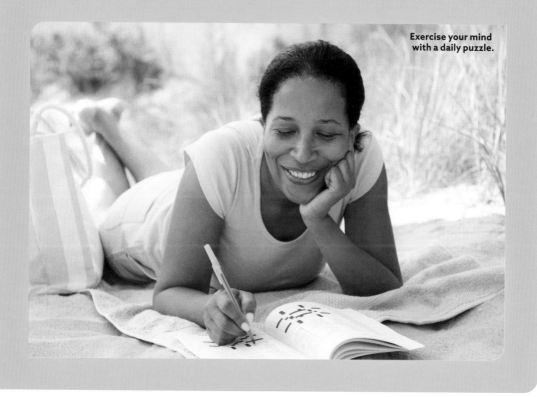

Exercise your mind with a daily puzzle.

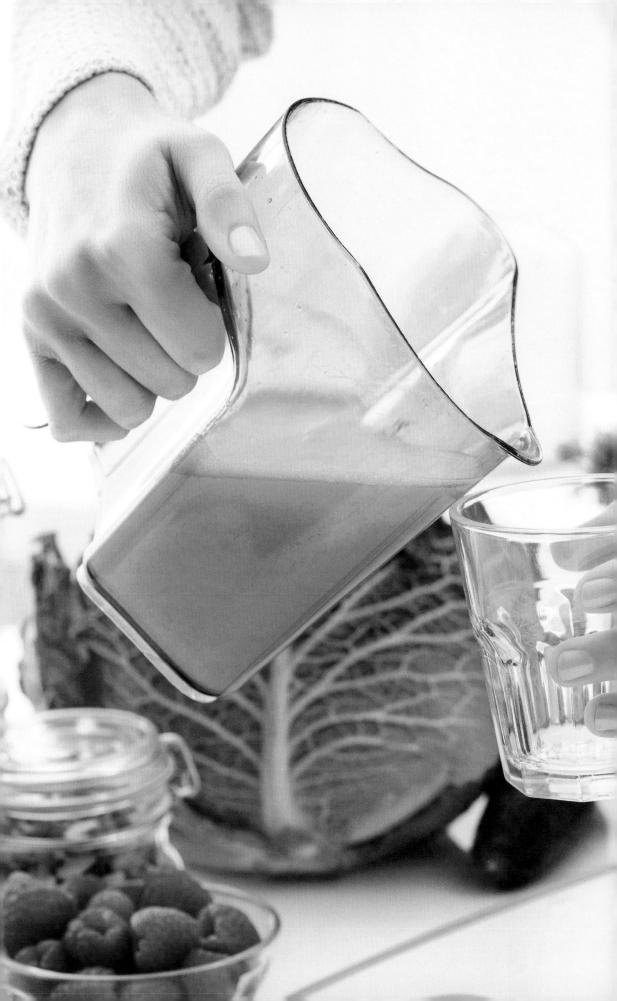

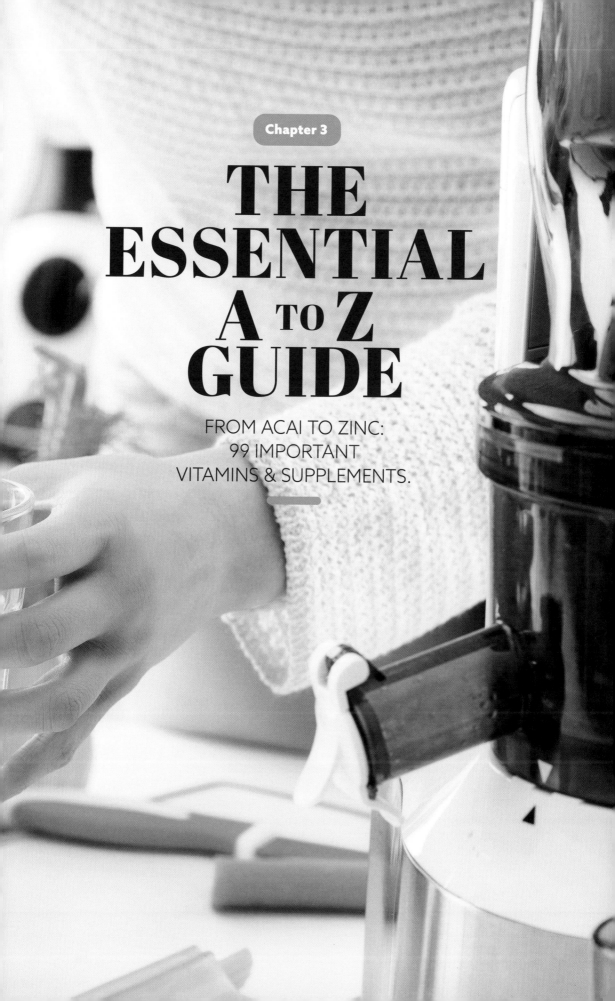

Chapter 3

THE ESSENTIAL A TO Z GUIDE

FROM ACAI TO ZINC:
99 IMPORTANT
VITAMINS & SUPPLEMENTS.

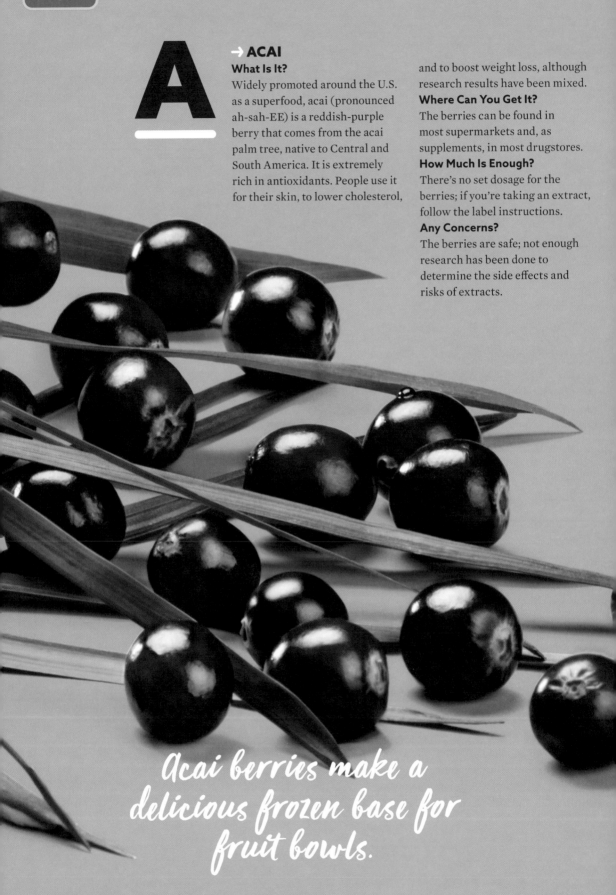

A

→ ACAI

What Is It?

Widely promoted around the U.S. as a superfood, acai (pronounced ah-sah-EE) is a reddish-purple berry that comes from the acai palm tree, native to Central and South America. It is extremely rich in antioxidants. People use it for their skin, to lower cholesterol, and to boost weight loss, although research results have been mixed.

Where Can You Get It?

The berries can be found in most supermarkets and, as supplements, in most drugstores.

How Much Is Enough?

There's no set dosage for the berries; if you're taking an extract, follow the label instructions.

Any Concerns?

The berries are safe; not enough research has been done to determine the side effects and risks of extracts.

Acai berries make a delicious frozen base for fruit bowls.

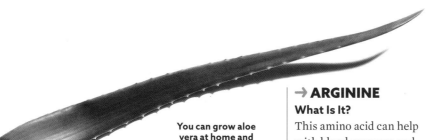

You can grow aloe vera at home and use the gel from the leaves.

→ ALOE VERA

What Is It?

Typically in gel form, aloe comes from a cactus-like plant that grows in hot, dry climates. It's most commonly used as an ointment for burns, sun damage and skin abrasions. But recent studies suggest it can also help with weight loss, if taken orally. Loaded with antioxidants, aloe is soothing to the digestive tract, according to some research.

Where Can You Get It?

The gel is widely available in drugstores, convenience stores and supermarkets.

How Much Is Enough?

For sunburns, applying aloe twice a day for six weeks is recommended. For weight loss, some people have taken 147 mg, twice a day, for a total of eight weeks.

Any Concerns?

High oral doses of aloe may cause side effects such as diarrhea, kidney problems, potassium loss, blood in urine, heart issues or muscle weakness. The plant may be unsafe for pregnant women and children under 12.

→ ARGININE

What Is It?

This amino acid can help with blood pressure and other heart conditions. The body uses it to make proteins.

Where Can You Get It?

Arginine can be found in meat, soy, whole grains, beans and dairy.

How Much Is Enough?

While there's no standard dose, studies suggest 2 to 3 grams, three times a day, may make sense.

Any Concerns?

There are a few potential side effects, such as nausea, cramps, diarrhea, allergic reactions and asthma symptoms. Also, if you have a medical condition—heart issues, cancer, liver or kidney problems or a bleeding disorder, for example— don't take arginine without talking to a doctor first.

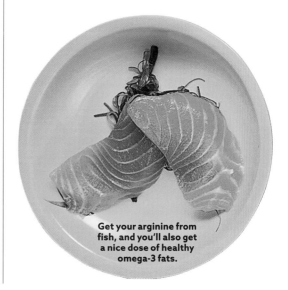

Get your arginine from fish, and you'll also get a nice dose of healthy omega-3 fats.

→ ASTRAGALUS

What Is It?

This herb is in the legume family. While there isn't a lot of research on it, some studies suggest it may stimulate the immune system and help control blood sugar in people with type 2 diabetes.

Where Can You Get It?

Most drugstores, in pill form or dried leaves.

How Much Is Enough?

The research isn't clear, but it typically comes in 500 mg capsules. Follow the label directions.

Any Concerns?

Since it stimulates the immune system, anyone with an autoimmune condition should avoid this herb.

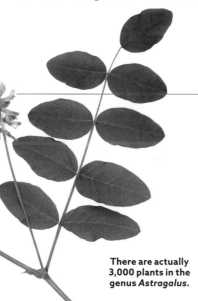

There are actually 3,000 plants in the genus *Astragalus*.

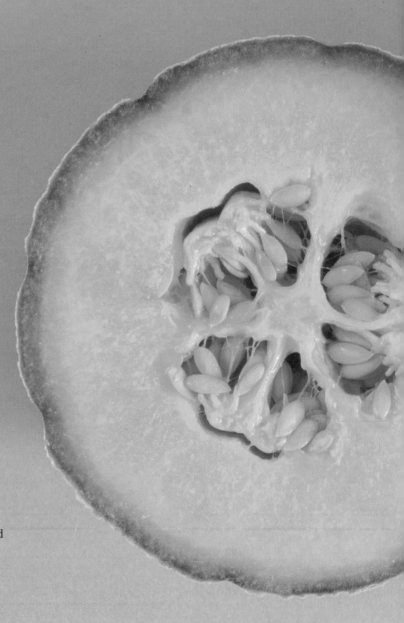

B

→ BETA-CAROTENE

What Is It?

This vitamin is part of a group of red, orange and yellow pigments called carotenoids. The body converts beta-carotene to vitamin A and it accounts for 50% of our A intake. It protects cells from damage and may protect against breast and ovarian cancers.

Where Can You Get It?

Beta-carotene can be found in fruits, vegetables and whole grains.

How Much Is Enough?

More research is needed to set an RDA for beta-carotene.

Any Concerns?

Most health authorities—including the American Cancer Society—recommend that you get beta-carotene from food only, as supplements might not offer the same benefits and may be dangerous if taken in high doses. Also, beta-carotene can be bad for smokers—it may increase the risk of colon, lung and prostate cancers.

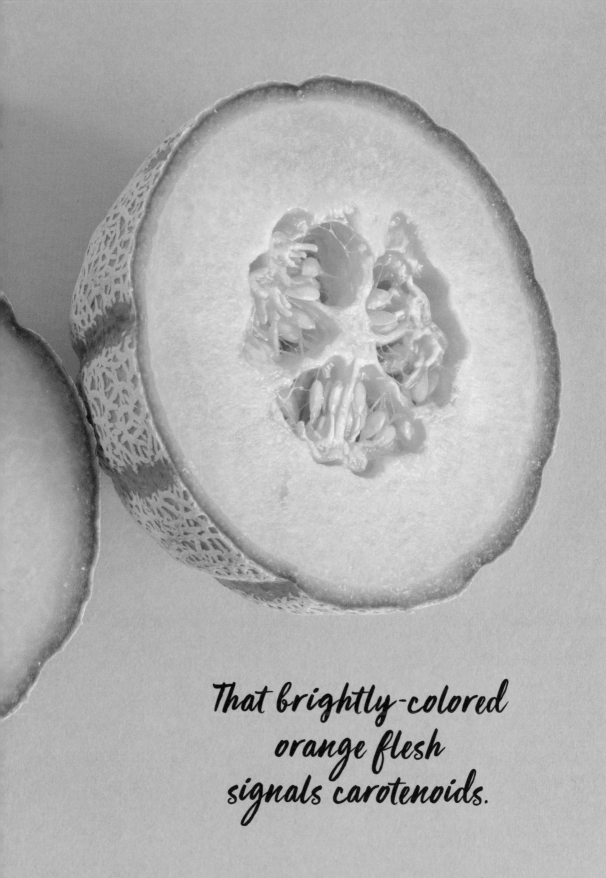

That brightly-colored
orange flesh
signals carotenoids.

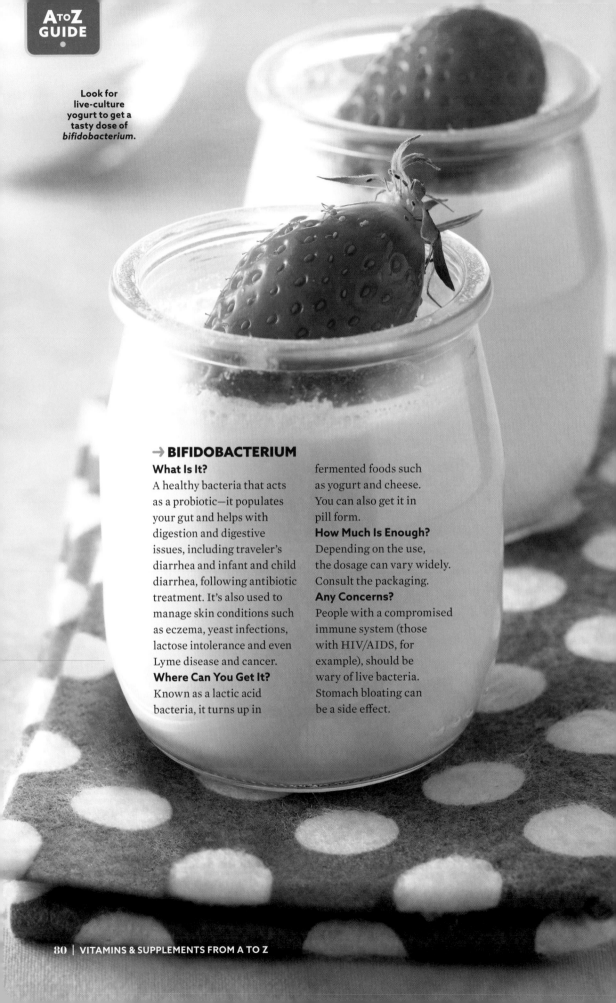

Look for live-culture yogurt to get a tasty dose of *bifidobacterium.*

→ BIFIDOBACTERIUM

What Is It?

A healthy bacteria that acts as a probiotic—it populates your gut and helps with digestion and digestive issues, including traveler's diarrhea and infant and child diarrhea, following antibiotic treatment. It's also used to manage skin conditions such as eczema, yeast infections, lactose intolerance and even Lyme disease and cancer.

Where Can You Get It?

Known as a lactic acid bacteria, it turns up in fermented foods such as yogurt and cheese. You can also get it in pill form.

How Much Is Enough?

Depending on the use, the dosage can vary widely. Consult the packaging.

Any Concerns?

People with a compromised immune system (those with HIV/AIDS, for example), should be wary of live bacteria. Stomach bloating can be a side effect.

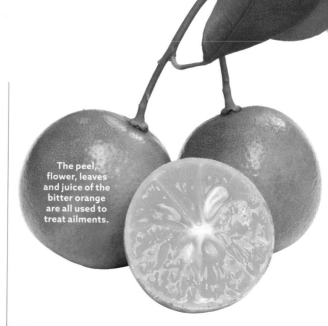

The peel, flower, leaves and juice of the bitter orange are all used to treat ailments.

→ BILBERRY

What Is It?
Healers use this plant's fruit and leaves to make medicine. Bilberry contains anthocyanins that can improve circulation; it can also tame mouth and throat irritation by reducing swelling. Military doctors gave it to British Air Force pilots in World War II to improve night vision, but research has since debunked that use.

Where Can You Get It?
It can be found in most drugstores.

How Much Is Enough?
Typically, 20 to 60 grams of dried, ripe berries daily. People also drink a type of tea made from 5–10 grams of the mashed berries.

Any Concerns?
It can interfere with diabetes medications; because it helps circulation, it should be avoided if you have surgery scheduled. As always, check with your doctor if you're considering taking bilberry.

→ BITTER ORANGE

What Is It?
Native to Southeast Asia, bitter orange has anti-fungal abilities; taken orally, it affects the nervous system.

Where Can You Get It?
Supplements and oils can be found in drugstores.

How Much Is Enough?
For treatment of fungal skin infections, apply pure oil of bitter orange once daily for one to three weeks.

Any Concerns?
Bitter orange may aggravate diabetes, high blood pressure, glaucoma and heart disease. It can also interfere with depression medication and may trigger seizures or anxiety.

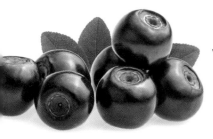

Bilberry may offer some vision benefits, including protection against glaucoma.

→ BIOTIN

What Is It?
Also known as B7, biotin is an important coenzyme that breaks down fats and carbohydrates. It's used primarily for mild depression, hair loss, hepatitis, brittle nails and neuropathy. While there is a good amount of evidence on the effectiveness of other B vitamins, researchers still don't know a lot about B7.

Where Can You Get It?
Liver, eggs, nuts, cauliflower and seeds.

How Much Is Enough?
There's no RDA for B7, but 30 mcg a day seems to be an adequate intake for adults 18 years and older.

Any Concerns?
Pregnant women should not go beyond 30 mcg. There's also some concern it may interact or interfere with the way your liver breaks down other medications. Discuss concerns with your doctor before taking biotin supplements.

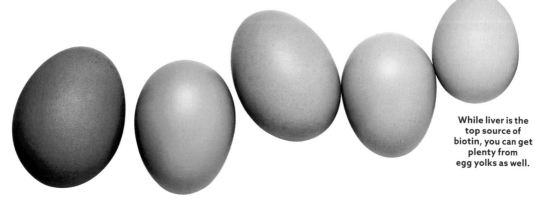

While liver is the top source of biotin, you can get plenty from egg yolks as well.

→ BLACK COHOSH

What Is It?

First introduced by Native Americans to European colonists, black cohosh contains many active substances, primarily in the roots, that act on the immune system and brain; it even has chemicals with estrogen-like properties. The herb has long been used to manage premenstrual syndrome (PMS), menopausal symptoms, migraines and arthritis.

Where Can You Get It?

It's available at most drugstores.

How Much Is Enough?

For the symptoms of menopause, 20 to 80 mg, once or twice daily.

Any Concerns?

The biggest risk for taking black cohosh is during pregnancy: Even though it has not been named the primary cause, it has been linked to miscarriage. It also might worsen existing breast cancer.

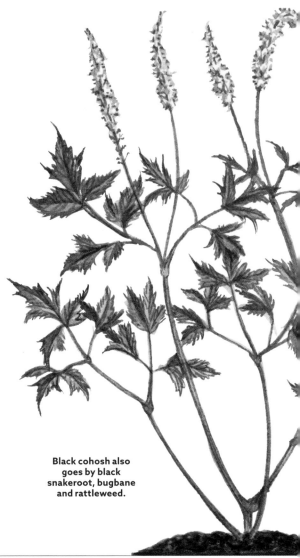

Black cohosh also goes by black snakeroot, bugbane and rattleweed.

→ BOVINE CARTILAGE

What Is It?

As you might guess, this cartilage comes from cows. Research indicates that it can reduce swelling and help wounds heal more quickly. People apply bovine cartilage topically to treat external hemorrhoids and rectal itching; it can also ease skin conditions such as acne, psoriasis and rashes (dermatitis) caused by poison oak and poison ivy.

Where Can You Get It?

You can find it in supplements and creams at most drugstores.

How Much Is Enough?

Doctors recommend a 5% cream for wounds and other skin conditions.

Any Concerns?

This cartilage is generally considered safe, but some people experience side effects such as diarrhea, nausea, swelling, local redness and itching.

There is concern that bovine cartilage could transmit mad cow disease. Avoid products from countries where that disease has been found.

→ BUTTERBUR

What Is It?

A plant with large woolly leaves found in North America, Europe and Asia, butterbur was originally used in the Middle Ages to combat plague and fever. Today, the roots of the butterbur plant are used medicinally to treat migraines, urinary tract symptoms, upset stomach and hay fever. Butterbur contains chemicals that can reduce swelling and alleviate spasms, although more research is needed to determine its effectiveness.

Where Can You Get It?

Butterbur products that contain extracts from the root, rhizome (underground stem) or leaves of the plant are available at drugstores.

How Much Is Enough?

In studies, people have taken 50 to 100 mg a day to treat migraines.

Any Concerns?

Unprocessed butterbur plant contains chemicals called pyrrolizidine alkaloids (PAs). PAs can cause liver damage, so only use butterbur products that have been processed to remove PAs and are labeled or certified as PA-free. Several studies, including a few with children and adolescents, have reported that PA-free butterbur products are safe and well tolerated when taken by mouth in recommended doses for up to 16 weeks. However, the safety of longer-term use has not been established.

Put the kibosh on that migraine.

To fully absorb calcium, you'll need vitamin D and other nutrients.

C

→ CALCIUM

What Is It?

This essential mineral's primary job in the body is to help keep your bones strong. But a small amount is put to use supporting your muscles, helping your blood clot and facilitating nerve communication.

Where Can You Get It?

Dairy, but it can also be found in leafy greens, seafood and legumes.

How Much Is Enough?

The RDA for adults starts at 1,000 mg; for women over 50, the RDA increases to 1,200 mg.

Any Concerns?

One recent study found taking more than 1,000 mg of calcium supplements a day was linked to a higher risk of cancer deaths. Doses above the RDA for calcium may also raise heart attack risk.

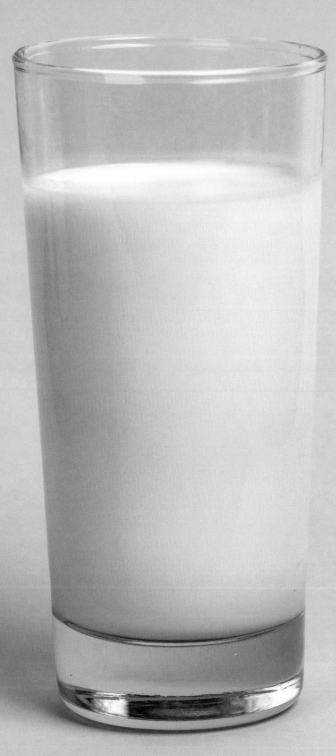

→ CAT'S CLAW

What Is It?

A vine with claw-like thorns, it's found in the Amazon rain forest and other tropical areas of Central and South America. The use of cat's claw dates back to the time of the Inca and it is believed to contain chemicals that stimulate the immune system. It is used today to combat viral infections, arthritis, Alzheimer's disease, cancer and other conditions. There are no conclusive studies to support its effectiveness.

Where Can You Get It?

The bark and root are used to make liquid extracts, capsules, tablets and tea, which are available at drugstores.

How Much Is Enough?

In research, people have taken 100 mg a day.

Any Concerns?

When taken in small amounts, few side effects have been reported; however, women who are pregnant or trying to get pregnant should avoid it.

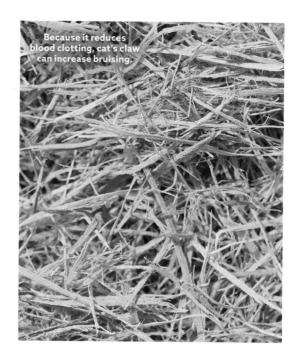
Because it reduces blood clotting, cat's claw can increase bruising.

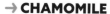

→ CHAMOMILE

What Is It?

Used for centuries, chamomile tea is relaxing and can help with falling asleep. There are two types of chamomile: German and Roman (or English). German chamomile has more research to support it; while both work for upset stomach, German chamomile can also be used topically to reduce swelling and fight bacteria.

Where Can You Get It?

You can buy the tea at supermarkets and the dried flower, liquid extract, creams and ointments at drugstores.

How Much Is Enough?

There is no RDA, but 1 milliliter (ml) in tea has been used to treat upset stomach.

Any Concerns?

If you are allergic to ragweed, you may not be able to use chamomile.

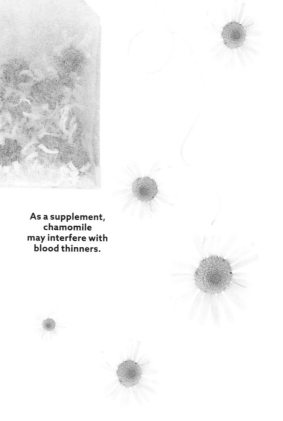

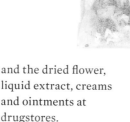
As a supplement, chamomile may interfere with blood thinners.

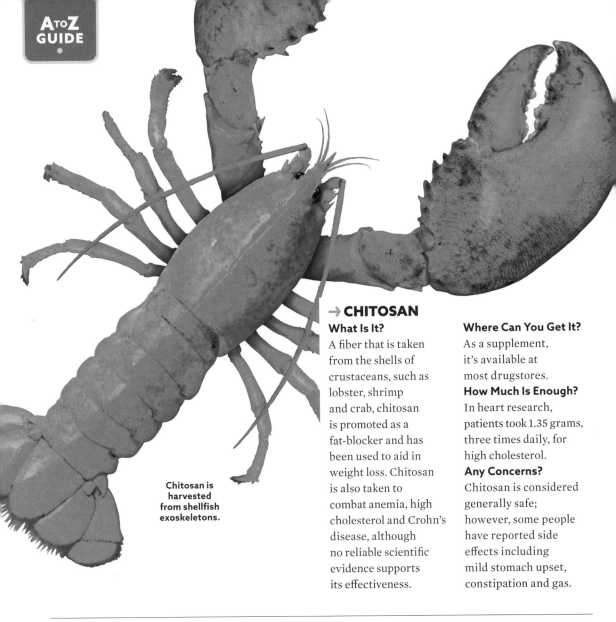

Chitosan is harvested from shellfish exoskeletons.

→ CHITOSAN

What Is It?

A fiber that is taken from the shells of crustaceans, such as lobster, shrimp and crab, chitosan is promoted as a fat-blocker and has been used to aid in weight loss. Chitosan is also taken to combat anemia, high cholesterol and Crohn's disease, although no reliable scientific evidence supports its effectiveness.

Where Can You Get It?

As a supplement, it's available at most drugstores.

How Much Is Enough?

In heart research, patients took 1.35 grams, three times daily, for high cholesterol.

Any Concerns?

Chitosan is considered generally safe; however, some people have reported side effects including mild stomach upset, constipation and gas.

→ CHOLINE

What Is It?

Very similar to B vitamins, choline is a nutrient produced by the liver that is involved in chemical reactions throughout the body. It is mainly given to people with liver disease who can't produce enough; however, people have also used it to treat asthma.

Where Can You Get It?

Choline can be found in the liver of other animals, but you can also get it from beans, broccoli, spinach, wheat germ and eggs.

How Much Is Enough?

The adequate intakes (AI) for adults are 550 mg per day for men and breastfeeding women; for pregnant women, 450 mg; for other women, 425 mg per day.

Any Concerns?

Don't overdo it: When people exceed the recommended amounts, they can have side effects such as sweating, a fishy body odor, GI distress, diarrhea or vomiting.

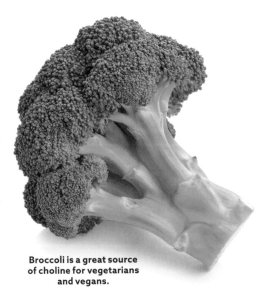

Broccoli is a great source of choline for vegetarians and vegans.

→ CHONDROITIN

What Is It?

Found in cartilage around joints in the body, chondroitin is usually manufactured from shark and cow cartilage. It may help with urinary tract infections, but its most popular and studied use is for osteoarthritis. Chondroitin seems to slow the breakdown of joint cartilage linked to arthritis.

Where Can You Get It?

As a supplement, at most drugstores.

How Much Is Enough?

For arthritis, 800–2,000 mg, taken daily as a single dose or in two or three divided doses.

Any Concerns?

Chondroitin is considered generally safe, but it may worsen asthma symptoms in some cases.

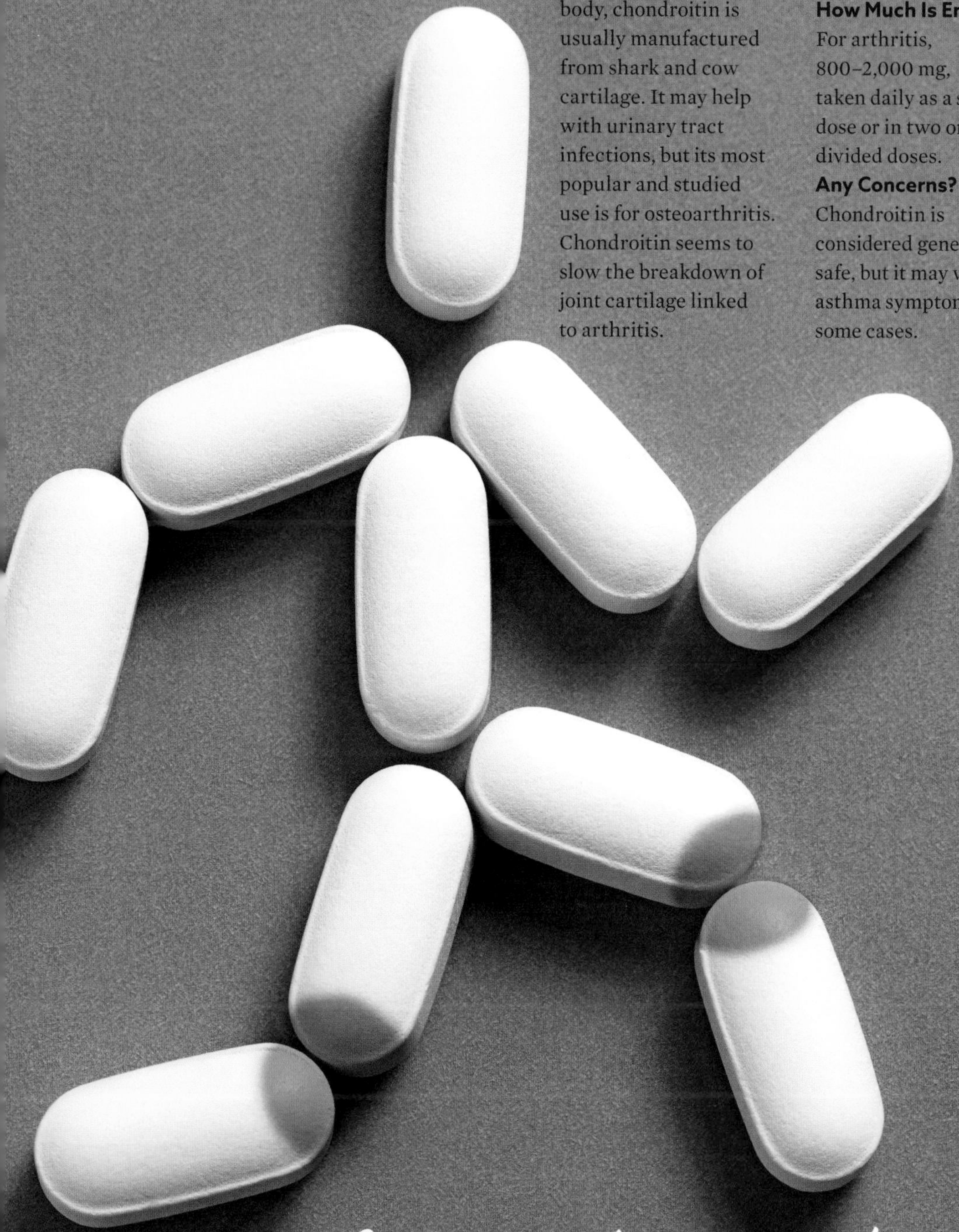

Some people report that chondroitin eases sore muscles.

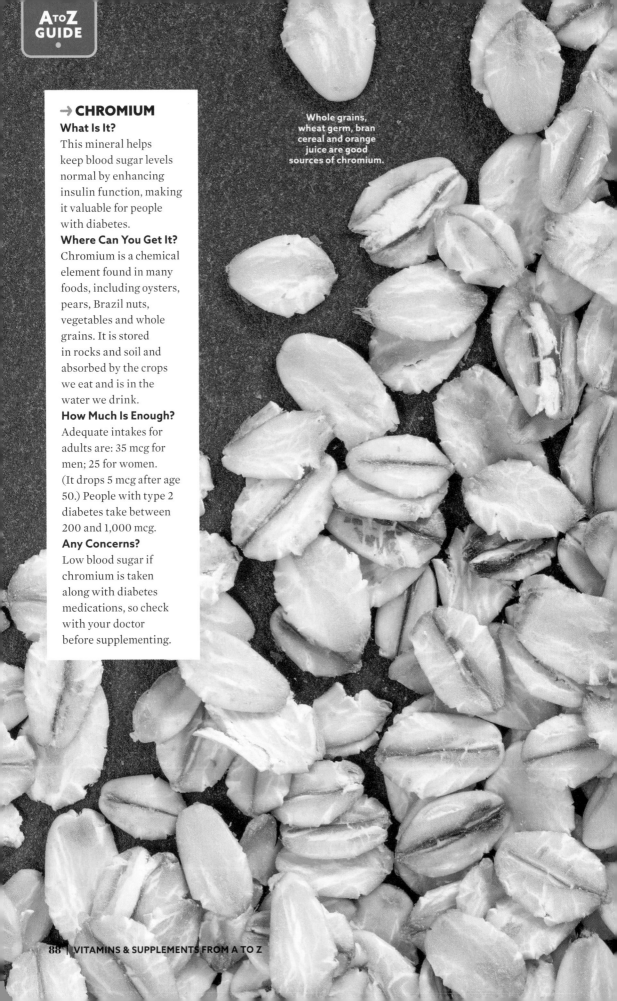

→ CHROMIUM

What Is It?

This mineral helps keep blood sugar levels normal by enhancing insulin function, making it valuable for people with diabetes.

Where Can You Get It?

Chromium is a chemical element found in many foods, including oysters, pears, Brazil nuts, vegetables and whole grains. It is stored in rocks and soil and absorbed by the crops we eat and is in the water we drink.

How Much Is Enough?

Adequate intakes for adults are: 35 mcg for men; 25 for women. (It drops 5 mcg after age 50.) People with type 2 diabetes take between 200 and 1,000 mcg.

Any Concerns?

Low blood sugar if chromium is taken along with diabetes medications, so check with your doctor before supplementing.

Whole grains, wheat germ, bran cereal and orange juice are good sources of chromium.

→ COENZYME Q10

What Is It?

This vitamin-like substance plays a role in vital chemical reactions throughout the body; people take it for disorders that limit energy production (mitochondrial disorders). It may also protect aging vision.

Where Can You Get It?

In organ meats and, in smaller amounts, in other meats and seafood.

How Much Is Enough?

Typically around 150–160 mg, or 1 mg per pound of body weight.

Any Concerns?

Few side effects, though some users reported an upset stomach. CoQ10 can lower blood sugar levels, so those with diabetes should avoid this supplement.

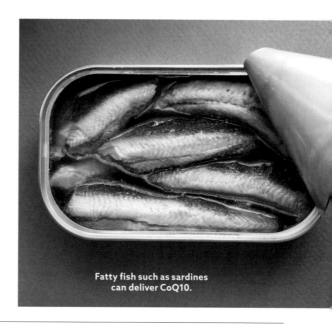

Fatty fish such as sardines can deliver CoQ10.

→ CONJUGATED LINOLEIC ACID (CLA)

What Is It?

Scientists believe this healthy fat may reduce body fat and improve immune function. It has been used for cancer, atherosclerosis, obesity, weight loss caused by chronic disease and for limiting food allergies.

Where Can You Get It?

Dairy products and beef are the major dietary sources of CLA, but it can also be made into supplements.

How Much Is Enough?

In studies, 1.8 to 7 grams daily have been given.

Any Concerns?

CLA is generally safe, but may cause upset stomach, diarrhea, nausea or fatigue.

CLA may be one of the reasons dairy has been linked to weight loss.

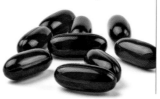

→ COPPER

What Is It?

This essential mineral is found in nearly every tissue of the body; it assists in making red blood cells, maintaining nerve cells and supporting the immune system.

Where Can You Get It?

Copper is found in many foods, such as shellfish, organ meats, leafy greens, certain nuts, cocoa and beans.

How Much Is Enough?

The adult RDA is 900 mcg.

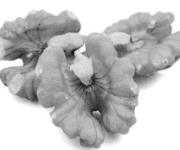

Walnuts are a safe— and healthy—way to get copper.

Any Concerns?

Copper is considered generally safe, but doses above the RDA can cause nausea, vomiting and, in rare cases, death.

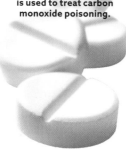

A true lifesaver: Cysteine is used to treat carbon monoxide poisoning.

→ CYSTEINE

What Is It?

This amino acid is found in the body, and it's a potent antioxidant. It is used for chest pain, bile duct blockage in infants, amyotrophic lateral sclerosis (ALS, aka Lou Gehrig's disease) and Alzheimer's disease.

Where Can You Get It?

Supplements are sold at most drugstores.

How Much Is Enough?

Around 600 mg per day.

Any Concerns?

Cysteine is considered generally safe; it may cause nausea, vomiting and diarrhea or constipation and, rarely, rashes, fever, headaches and liver issues.

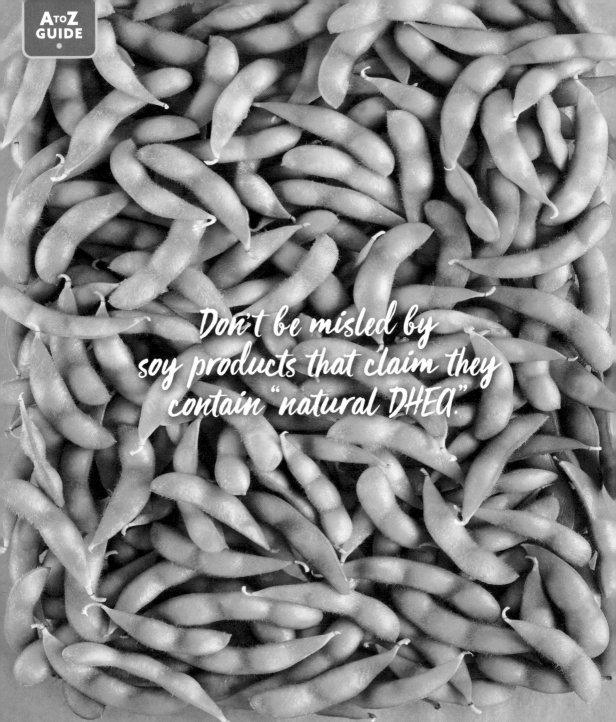

Don't be misled by soy products that claim they contain "natural DHEA."

D

→ DHEA

What Is It?

DHEA (dehydroepi-androsterone), is a hormone produced in the adrenal glands and assists in generating testosterone and estrogen. Related to growth hormone, DHEA is taken as an anti-aging therapy; it may also help with osteoporosis and depression.

Where Can You Get It?

It needs to be synthesized: Although it's in soy and wild yams, the body cannot convert this version to increase its own DHEA levels.

How Much Is Enough?

Depending on the use, between 30 and 450 mg a day.

Any Concerns?

Large doses or long-term use can trigger dangerous side effects. Take it only under a doctor's supervision.

E

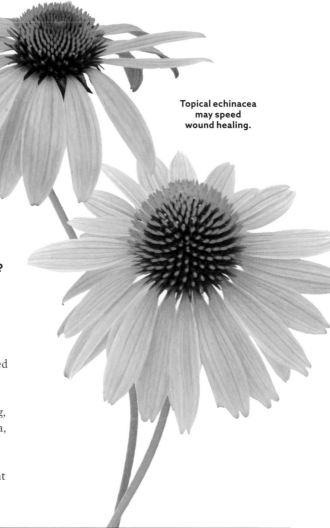

Topical echinacea may speed wound healing.

→ ECHINACEA

What Is It?
Also known as purple coneflower, echinacea is a flowering plant used mainly to boost the immune system. It can be taken as a dietary supplement to battle the common cold and other infections.

Where Can You Get It?
Echinacea is most commonly found in capsule or tablet form; however, the roots, leaves and flowers can be used either fresh or dried in teas and juices, as well as in external uses.

How Much Is Enough?
Use an extract of 5 ml, twice a day, for 10 days to treat the common cold.

Any Concerns?
Echinacea is considered generally safe, but some people report fever, nausea, vomiting, stomach pain, diarrhea, sore throat, headache, dizziness, insomnia, disorientation and joint and muscle aches.

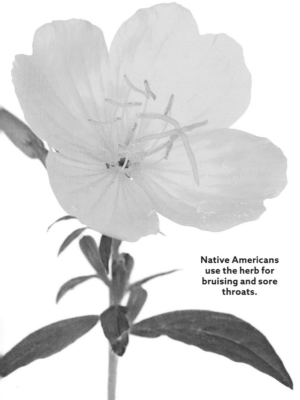

Native Americans use the herb for bruising and sore throats.

→ EVENING PRIMROSE OIL

What Is It?
Used by Native Americans for medicinal purposes, evening primrose oil is now used primarily to treat skin disorders, such as eczema, psoriasis and acne. It can also treat a number of conditions including premenstrual syndrome (PMS), menopausal symptoms and rheumatoid arthritis.

Where Can You Get It?
It's extracted from the seeds of the evening primrose plant and sold in capsule form.

How Much Is Enough?
There is no RDA, but 3–4 grams per day have been used for breast pain.

Any Concerns?
When taken in short intervals, evening primrose oil is generally considered safe for most people; some side effects that have been reported include headaches and upset stomach. Results on the safety of taking evening primrose oil for long periods of time are unclear, so consult your doctor before using.

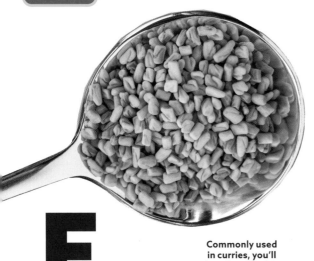

Commonly used in curries, you'll love fenugreek's maple scent.

F

→ FENUGREEK

What Is It?
The plant looks like clover; the seeds can be helpful in managing blood sugar for diabetics. New moms have used the herb to stimulate milk production during breastfeeding. Although the research is preliminary, fenugreek has shown promise as a dressing for wounds and for eczema.

Where Can You Get It?
Fenugreek leaves and seeds can be found in health food stores; it's also sold in capsules, teas and creams.

How Much Is Enough?
In studies, 5–50 grams of seed powder, taken with meals twice a day, have been used for diabetes.

Any Concerns?
Pregnant women should avoid it; it may trigger uterine contractions. Side effects include diarrhea and other mild stomach upset; a sweet, maple smell to urine, breast milk and perspiration; and a worsening of asthma.

→ FEVERFEW

What Is It?
Historically used to treat fevers, headaches, constipation, diarrhea and dizziness, scientists have found that feverfew may be most effective for preventing migraines. Feverfew leaves contain many different chemicals, including one called parthenolide, which has been shown to decrease factors in the body that may cause migraine headaches.

Where Can You Get It?
Supplements can be found in most drugstores.

How Much Is Enough?
Try 50–150 mg of feverfew for four months.

Any Concerns?
No serious side effects.

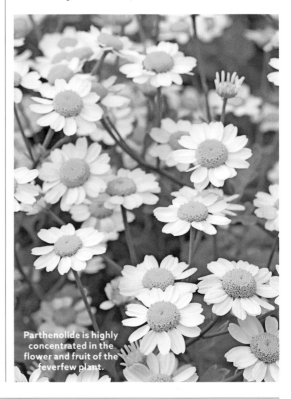

Parthenolide is highly concentrated in the flower and fruit of the feverfew plant.

→ FISH OIL

What Is It?
There's evidence that this popular supplement, extracted from fatty fish, can protect against heart disease, smooth mood problems and help kids with attention-deficit/hyperactivity disorder (ADHD). A lot of the benefit of fish oil seems to come from the omega-3 fatty acids that it contains. Omega-3s are essential nutrients that may boost brain health and prevent heart disease, among other attributes.

Where Can You Get It?
By eating cold-water fatty fish such as salmon, tuna and sardines or by taking supplements, which can be found in most drugstores.

How Much Is Enough?
The American Heart Association OKs up to 3 grams of fish oil daily.

Any Concerns?
A fishy taste in your mouth, fishy breath, upset stomach, loose stools, nausea. More than 3 grams daily interferes with clotting.

Big benefits, for such a small capsule.

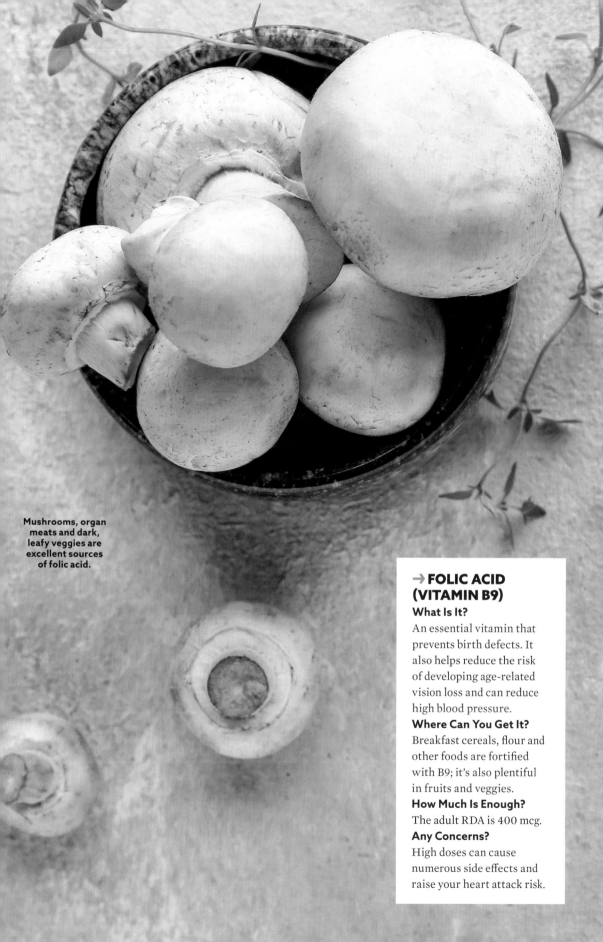

Mushrooms, organ meats and dark, leafy veggies are excellent sources of folic acid.

→ FOLIC ACID (VITAMIN B9)

What Is It?

An essential vitamin that prevents birth defects. It also helps reduce the risk of developing age-related vision loss and can reduce high blood pressure.

Where Can You Get It?

Breakfast cereals, flour and other foods are fortified with B9; it's also plentiful in fruits and veggies.

How Much Is Enough?

The adult RDA is 400 mcg.

Any Concerns?

High doses can cause numerous side effects and raise your heart attack risk.

G

→ GARLIC

What Is It?

This bulb is used to reduce cholesterol and blood pressure, boost immunity and prevent cancer and other diseases. The active ingredient seems to be a chemical called allicin.

Where Can You Get It?

You can find garlic supplements at most drugstores.

How Much Is Enough?

A common dose is 300 mg a day.

Any Concerns?

Mild side effects may include bad breath and body odor, heartburn and upset stomach.

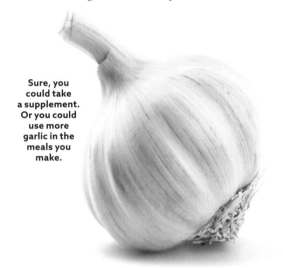

Sure, you could take a supplement. Or you could use more garlic in the meals you make.

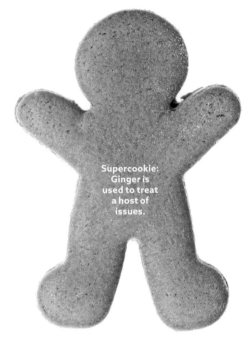

Supercookie: Ginger is used to treat a host of issues.

→ GINGER

What Is It?

This root is widely used as a flavoring or fragrance in foods, beverages and cosmetics. Ginger is considered an adaptogen and has been recommended for immunity, energy and other conditions. Now ginger is mainly used for nausea during pregnancy, for motion sickness and after chemotherapy and surgery.

Where Can You Get It?

Ginger root can be found in the produce section of most grocery stores or purchased as powder or capsules.

How Much Is Enough?

Typically 1–2 grams a day.

Any Concerns?

As a spice, it's safe. People report mild abdominal discomfort, heartburn, diarrhea and gas.

→ GINKGO

What Is It?

Ginkgo is a large tree native to Asia. The leaves and seeds have been cultivated for centuries for medicinal purposes. Ginkgo is taken to increase blood flow to the brain and has been useful in treating Alzheimer's, chronic headaches, dizziness and ringing in the ears.

Where Can You Get It?

Tablets, capsules, extracts and teas are widely available.

How Much Is Enough?

Start with a dosage of not more than 120 mg per day.

Any Concerns?

Side effects of ginkgo include headache, stomach upset and allergic skin reactions.

How old is ginkgo? Dinosaurs sought shade under these leaves!

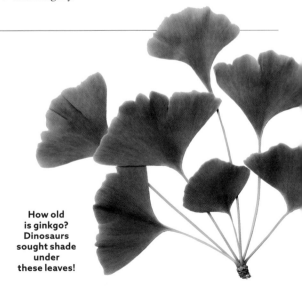

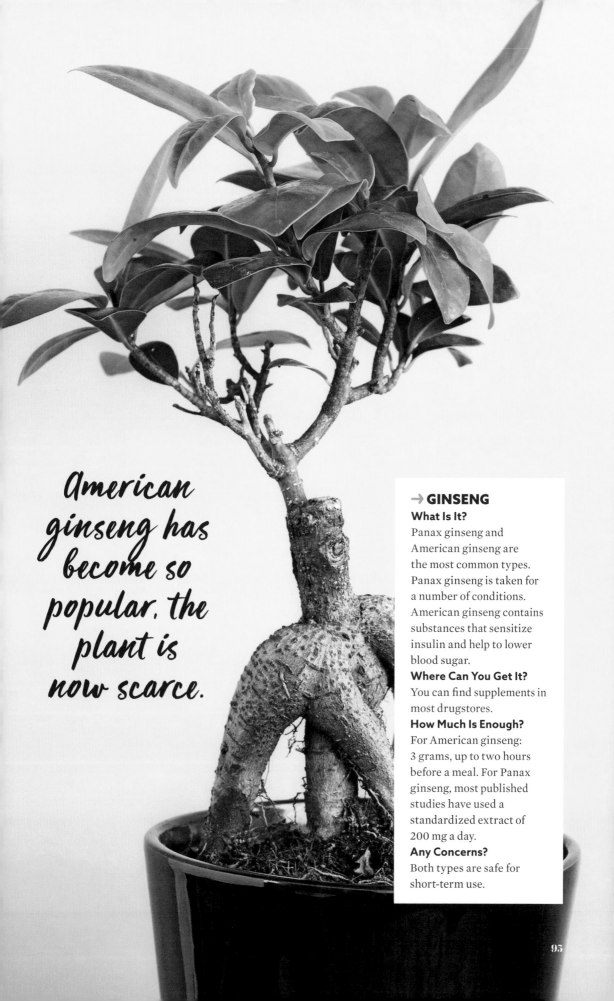

American ginseng has become so popular, the plant is now scarce.

→ GINSENG

What Is It?
Panax ginseng and American ginseng are the most common types. Panax ginseng is taken for a number of conditions. American ginseng contains substances that sensitize insulin and help to lower blood sugar.

Where Can You Get It?
You can find supplements in most drugstores.

How Much Is Enough?
For American ginseng: 3 grams, up to two hours before a meal. For Panax ginseng, most published studies have used a standardized extract of 200 mg a day.

Any Concerns?
Both types are safe for short-term use.

→ GLUCOMANNAN

What Is It?

A dietary fiber derived from the konjac plant, glucomannan has been used to treat weight loss, diabetes, constipation, high cholesterol, high blood pressure and various stomach conditions. Studies have shown it can help ease constipation and slow the absorption of sugar in the stomach to control sugar levels in diabetics.

Where Can You Get It?

In powders and capsules, in most drugstores; and in shirataki noodles at grocery stores.

How Much Is Enough?

Depending on the usage, the dose can vary, though many people start at around 2 grams daily. Follow label directions or check with your doctor.

Any Concerns?

Research has shown that the tablet form of glucomannan may cause blockages of the throat or intestines; take it under the supervision of a doctor. Also, glucomannan might interfere with your blood sugar control during surgery and shortly after. If you are scheduled for surgery, stop using glucomannan at least two weeks beforehand.

Glucomannan can help you stay regular.

→ GLUCOSAMINE

What Is It?
Your body produces this amino sugar, but more could offer benefits. Glucosamine sulfate is the type most studied. People take glucosamine sulfate orally to treat osteoarthritis.

Where Can You Get It?
Harvested from shells of shellfish or synthesized, you can find glucosamine sulfate supplements in most drugstores.

How Much Is Enough?
When used for treating osteoarthritis, the dose is 500 mg of glucosamine three times a day; some research recommends combining it with 400 mg of chondroitin two to three times daily.

Any Concerns?
Glucosamine sulfate can cause mild side effects including nausea, diarrhea and constipation—but scientists say it's generally safe for consumption.

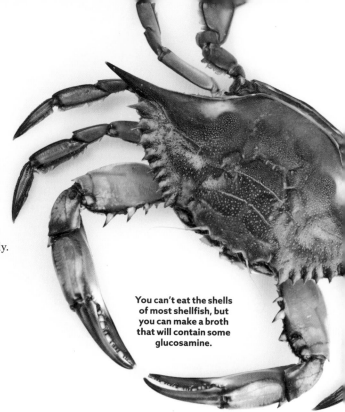

You can't eat the shells of most shellfish, but you can make a broth that will contain some glucosamine.

→ GLUTATHIONE

What Is It?
A substance produced naturally in the liver; your body uses it to build tissue and make chemicals and proteins. It may be most effective for reducing the side effects of chemotherapy treatments for cancer.

Where Can You Get It?
It's in sulfur-rich foods such as garlic, onions and cruciferous vegetables such as broccoli and cabbage. You can also find supplements at most drugstores.

How Much Is Enough?
There is no recommended intake for glutathione, as it is mainly used intravenously (IV) by doctors to treat patients going through chemotherapy.

Any Concerns?
Possible side effects are not yet known for this substance.

Combined with papaya, glutathione can be found in soaps used to reduce age spots and freckles.

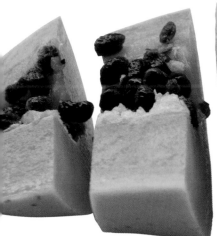

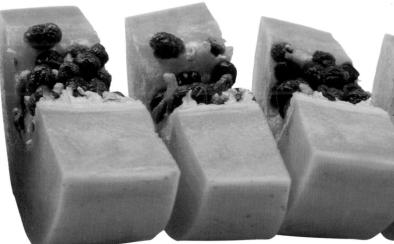

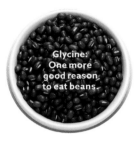

→ GLYCINE

What Is It?

This amino acid can be produced in your body—no help needed. Glycine is involved in the transmission of chemical signals in the brain, so there is interest in trying it for schizophrenia and improving memory. Some researchers think glycine may have a role in cancer prevention, because it seems to interfere with the blood supply needed by certain tumors. However, there has not been enough research done at this time to confirm these findings.

Where Can You Get It?

The primary sources for glycine are protein-rich foods, including meat, fish, dairy and legumes.

How Much Is Enough?

For schizophrenia, it has been used in doses ranging from 0.4 to 0.8 grams per kilogram (2.2 pounds) of body weight daily. It usually starts at 4 grams daily and is increased 4 grams per day until an effective dose is reached.

Any Concerns?

Glycine seems to be safe for most people when taken by mouth or applied to the skin. A few people have reported nausea, vomiting, stomach upset and drowsiness.

→ GOLDENSEAL

What Is It?

Overharvesting and loss of habitat have decreased the availability of wild goldenseal, but it's now grown commercially in the United States, especially in the Blue Ridge Mountains. People take it to treat colds and other respiratory tract infections, ulcers, and digestive upsets such as diarrhea and constipation. (It has also gained notoriety for supposedly masking illegal drugs in urine tests; it doesn't work, though.)

Where Can You Get It?

Goldenseal supplements can be found in most drugstores.

How Much Is Enough?

The appropriate dose depends on factors like the user's age and health; follow the dosing directions listed on product labels.

Any Concerns?

There isn't much reliable information on the safety of goldenseal. However, research suggests pregnant or breastfeeding women should avoid it; don't give it to infants.

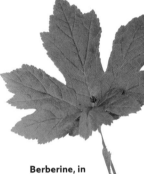

Berberine, in goldenseal, has antibacterial properties.

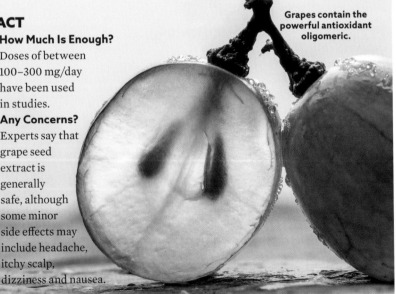

Grapes contain the powerful antioxidant oligomeric.

→ GRAPE SEED EXTRACT

What Is It?

People have been using grapes, grape leaves and sap for health, dating back to ancient Greece, but grape seed extract wasn't developed until the 1970s. It is used to help circulation, promote wound healing and reduce inflammation.

Where Can You Get It?

In capsules and tablets and as a liquid in drugstores.

How Much Is Enough?

Doses of between 100–300 mg/day have been used in studies.

Any Concerns?

Experts say that grape seed extract is generally safe, although some minor side effects may include headache, itchy scalp, dizziness and nausea.

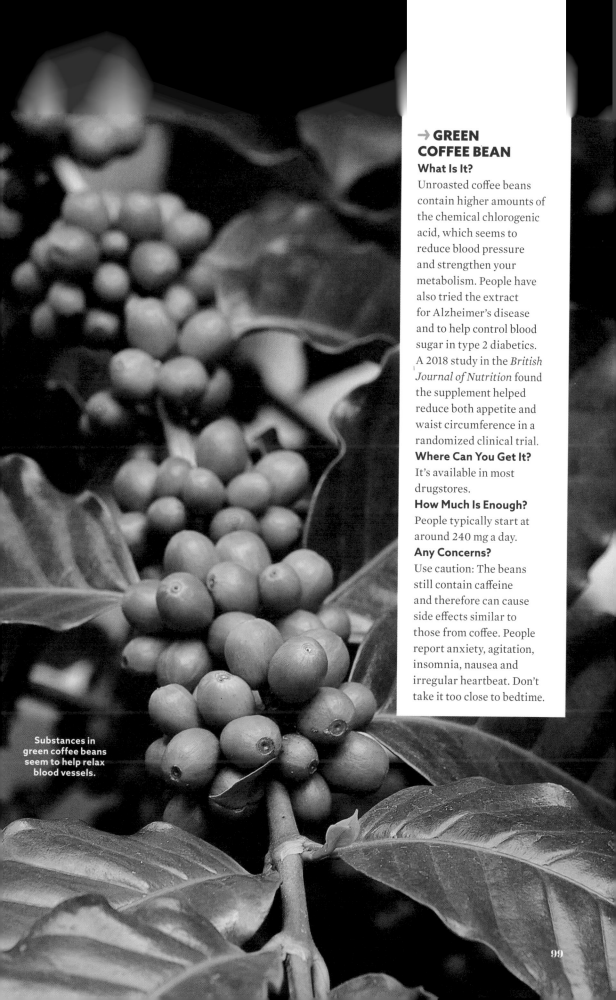

→ GREEN COFFEE BEAN

What Is It?

Unroasted coffee beans contain higher amounts of the chemical chlorogenic acid, which seems to reduce blood pressure and strengthen your metabolism. People have also tried the extract for Alzheimer's disease and to help control blood sugar in type 2 diabetics. A 2018 study in the *British Journal of Nutrition* found the supplement helped reduce both appetite and waist circumference in a randomized clinical trial.

Where Can You Get It?

It's available in most drugstores.

How Much Is Enough?

People typically start at around 240 mg a day.

Any Concerns?

Use caution: The beans still contain caffeine and therefore can cause side effects similar to those from coffee. People report anxiety, agitation, insomnia, nausea and irregular heartbeat. Don't take it too close to bedtime.

Substances in green coffee beans seem to help relax blood vessels.

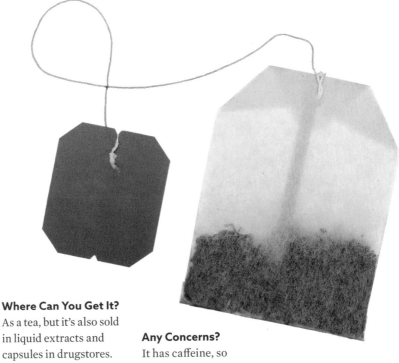

→ GREEN TEA

What Is It?

Extracted from the plant *Camellia sinensis*, green tea is used around the world to improve mental alertness and digestion, relieve headaches, promote weight loss and lower cholesterol. Research also shows that drinking green tea may be linked to preventing Parkinson's disease. The FDA has approved it as a prescription treatment for genital warts.

Where Can You Get It?

As a tea, but it's also sold in liquid extracts and capsules in drugstores.

How Much Is Enough?

Most people drink 2.5 cups for weight loss. As a supplement for cholesterol, people start at 150 mg, twice a day. For other uses, consult the product label.

Any Concerns?

It has caffeine, so the usual cautions apply. Taken long term or in high doses, sleeplessness, agitation, headache, nervousness, irritability, diarrhea or irregular heartbeat could result.

For best results, steep green tea two to three minutes.

→ GUAR GUM

What Is It?

This fiber can treat both diarrhea and constipation. How? It regulates the moisture, both soaking up excess liquid and softening the stool. Studies show it may also lower cholesterol and treat high blood pressure.

Where Can You Get It?

In supplements, sold at most drugstores.

How Much Is Enough?

About 15 grams per day is a common dosage.

Any Concerns?

Guar gum is safe, but side effects can include temporary diarrhea and excess gas.

Drink lots of water when taking guar gum to avoid developing a blockage.

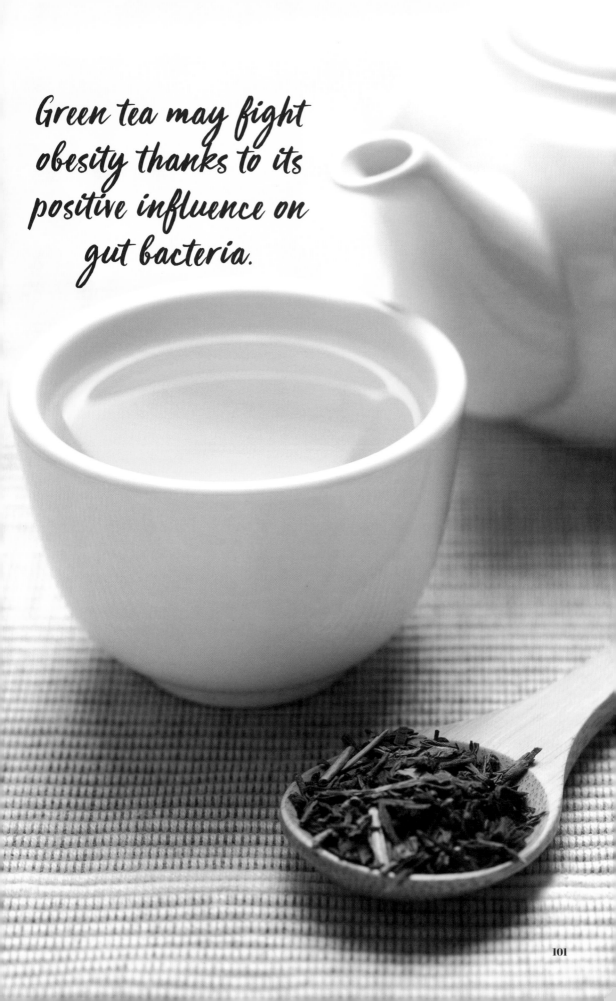

Green tea may fight obesity thanks to its positive influence on gut bacteria.

Research suggests hawthorn may be effective for treating anxiety.

H

→ HAWTHORN

What Is It?

This flowering shrub or tree is in the rose family. It's native to Europe and grows in temperate regions throughout the world. Historically, it's been used for heart, kidney and digestive issues.

Where Can You Get It?

In capsules, tablets or liquids in most drugstores.

How Much Is Enough?

Specific products have been used in doses of 160 to 1,800 mg, divided up and taken at two to three different times daily.

Any Concerns?

Some research suggests it may be linked to heart failure. Check with your doctor before using.

→ HOODIA

What Is It?

This flowering cactus-like plant is used by South African San (Bushmen) to ward off hunger during long hunts. It grows in the Kalahari Desert in Africa, and a chemical in hoodia called P57 does seem to suppress appetite—although research studies to date have been inconclusive.

Where Can You Get It?

Hoodia is available as liquids, powders, tablets and capsules at most drugstores.

How Much Is Enough?

Follow dosing instructions on the label.

Any Concerns?

Avoid if you have a condition such as diabetes, heart disease or high blood pressure.

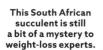

This South African succulent is still a bit of a mystery to weight-loss experts.

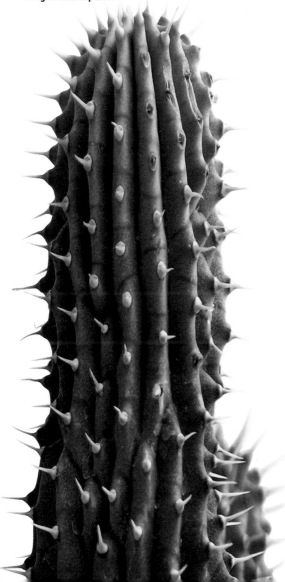

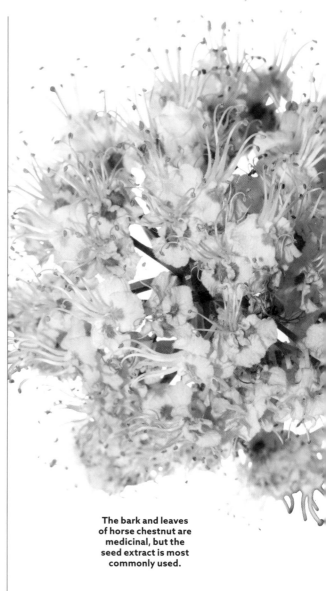

The bark and leaves of horse chestnut are medicinal, but the seed extract is most commonly used.

→ HORSE CHESTNUT

What Is It?

The horse chestnut plant's seeds and leaves contain a substance that thins the blood. Research shows the seed extract can treat chronic venous insufficiency and may have a cancer-fighting effect.

Where Can You Get It?

It's found in most drugstores.

How Much Is Enough?

For circulation, 300 mg of seed extract containing 50 mg of the active ingredient, aescin, twice daily is recommended.

Any Concerns?

Do not eat raw horse chestnut— it is dangerous. A standardized seed extract is safe.

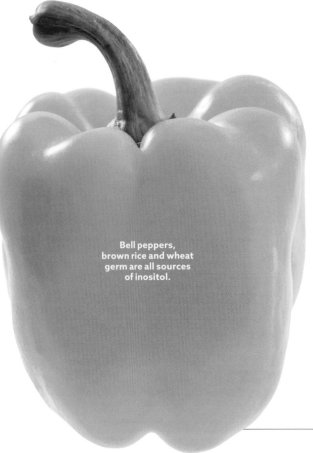

Bell peppers, brown rice and wheat germ are all sources of inositol.

I

→ INOSITOL

What Is It?

Research suggests this vitamin-like substance might help with conditions such as depression, obsessive-compulsive disorder, Alzheimer's disease, polycystic ovary syndrome and pain relief. It may also help with high blood pressure and cholesterol.

Where Can You Get It?

Oats, bran, almonds and walnuts contain high amounts of inositol, as do cantaloupe and all citrus fruits, other than lemons. It is available in supplement form at many drugstores.

How Much Is Enough?

For conditions such as panic disorder, depression and OCD, use 18 grams per day for three months.

Any Concerns?

Inositol is safe. Mild side effects such as nausea and excessive gas may occur.

→ IODINE

What Is It?

An essential element, we need iodine to make thyroid hormones and control metabolism. Since our bodies do not produce iodine, we must get it from our diet or supplements.

Where Can You Get It?

Salt that has been iodized is your best source. You can also get iodine from seaweed, fish (such as cod and tuna), dairy products such as milk and yogurt and grains such as breads and cereals.

How Much Is Enough?

For adults, 150 mcg a day.

Any Concerns?

Consuming large amounts is unsafe and can lead to thyroid problems; when used directly on the skin, it can cause irritation.

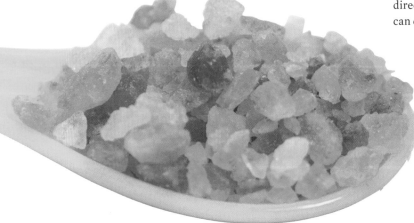

If you prefer sea salt over table salt, look for an iodized version.

Getting your iron from foods such as beans and meat may be your safest bet.

→ IRON

What Is It?

An essential mineral, iron helps your red blood cells deliver oxygen to the body and get rid of carbon monoxide. Iron deficiency can lead to anemia; symptoms include fatigue, dizziness, headache and pale skin. Iron may also be used to treat attention-deficit/hyperactivity disorder (ADHD) and for improving athletic performance.

Where Can You Get It?

There are many iron-rich foods. Animal sources—such as lean beef, turkey, chicken and oysters—provide more iron than plants, although beans, lentils, dark-green leafy vegetables and cashews are all good sources. Iron is also available in supplement form at most drugstores.

How Much Is Enough?

The adult RDA is 8 mg a day for men ages 19 and older and women ages 51 and older. For women 19 to 50 years, the RDA is 18 mg a day.

Any Concerns?

Getting too much iron is extremely dangerous, especially for children.

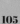

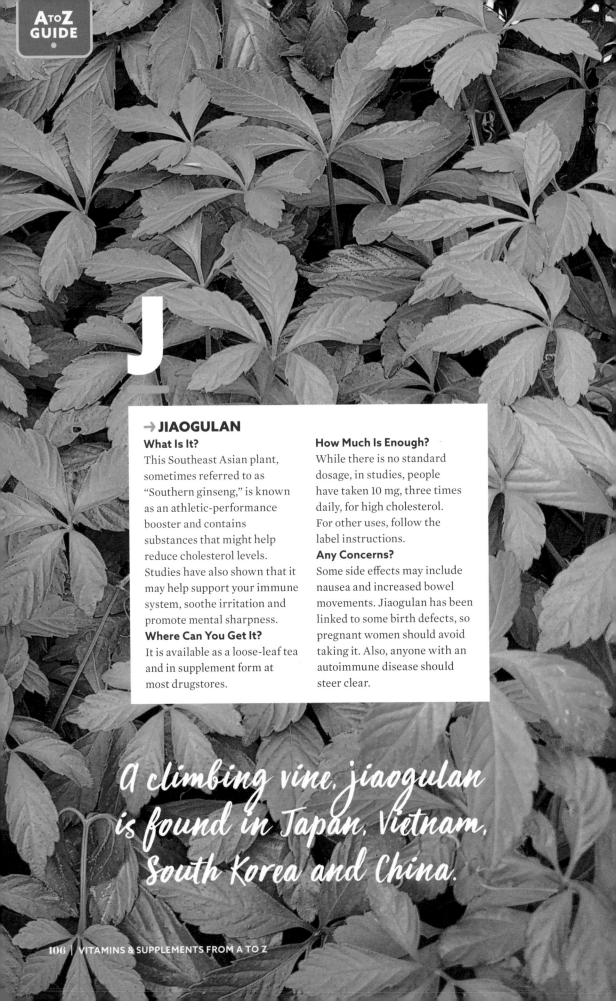

J

→ JIAOGULAN

What Is It?

This Southeast Asian plant, sometimes referred to as "Southern ginseng," is known as an athletic-performance booster and contains substances that might help reduce cholesterol levels. Studies have also shown that it may help support your immune system, soothe irritation and promote mental sharpness.

Where Can You Get It?

It is available as a loose-leaf tea and in supplement form at most drugstores.

How Much Is Enough?

While there is no standard dosage, in studies, people have taken 10 mg, three times daily, for high cholesterol. For other uses, follow the label instructions.

Any Concerns?

Some side effects may include nausea and increased bowel movements. Jiaogulan has been linked to some birth defects, so pregnant women should avoid taking it. Also, anyone with an autoimmune disease should steer clear.

A climbing vine, jiaogulan is found in Japan, Vietnam, South Korea and China.

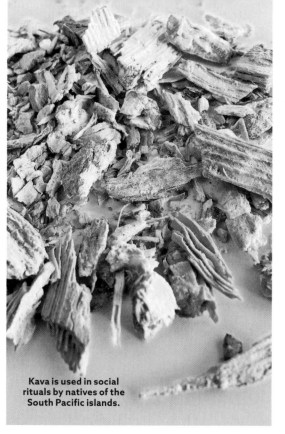

Kava is used in social rituals by natives of the South Pacific islands.

K

→ KAVA

What Is It?

A beverage or extract made from a plant native to the Pacific Islands, kava relaxes the brain and other parts of the central nervous system and has been used as a way to lower anxiety.

Where Can You Get It?

The root and stem of the plant are used to make drinks; they're also made into extracts, capsules and tablets. You can find these products in most drugstores.

How Much Is Enough?

Follow the package directions.

Any Concerns?

Kava may cause severe liver damage. Take only under a doctor's supervision.

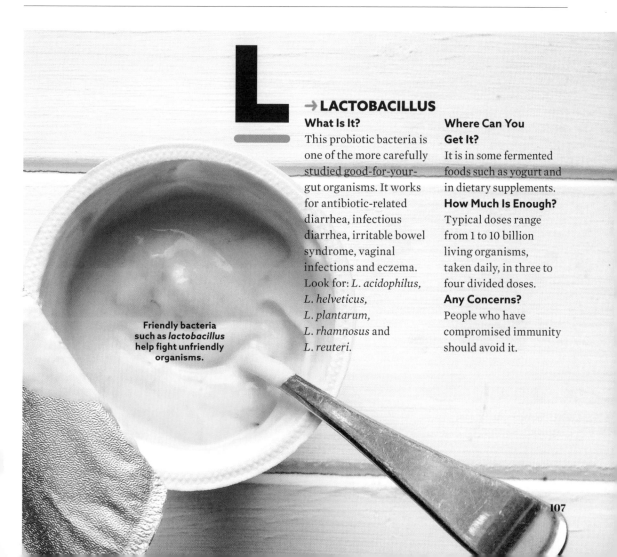

Friendly bacteria such as *lactobacillus* help fight unfriendly organisms.

L

→ LACTOBACILLUS

What Is It?

This probiotic bacteria is one of the more carefully studied good-for-your-gut organisms. It works for antibiotic-related diarrhea, infectious diarrhea, irritable bowel syndrome, vaginal infections and eczema. Look for: *L. acidophilus, L. helveticus, L. plantarum, L. rhamnosus* and *L. reuteri.*

Where Can You Get It?

It is in some fermented foods such as yogurt and in dietary supplements.

How Much Is Enough?

Typical doses range from 1 to 10 billion living organisms, taken daily, in three to four divided doses.

Any Concerns?

People who have compromised immunity should avoid it.

→ LAVENDER

What Is It?

This herb and its oil have long been used to treat anxiety, depression and insomnia, as well as relieve gastrointestinal problems. Research has shown lavender oil to be an effective tool in treating hair loss when rubbed on the scalp in combination with other oils, including cedarwood, thyme and rosemary. Therapeutic-grade lavender can be used to clean cuts and treat bruises and skin irritations.

Where Can You Get It?

The flower and the oil of lavender are used in supplements, and can be found in most drugstores.

How Much Is Enough?

The recommended dosage for hair loss is three drops, or 108 mg, of lavender oil in a mixture with other herbs.

Any Concerns?

Some people report skin irritation. The oil may be poisonous if taken by mouth; extracts may cause stomach upset, joint pain or headache.

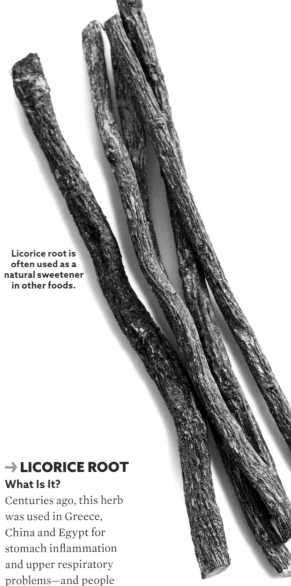

Licorice root is often used as a natural sweetener in other foods.

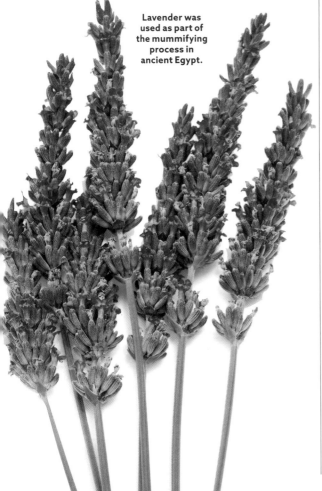

Lavender was used as part of the mummifying process in ancient Egypt.

→ LICORICE ROOT

What Is It?

Centuries ago, this herb was used in Greece, China and Egypt for stomach inflammation and upper respiratory problems—and people still use it for those complaints today, as well as for menopausal symptoms and bacterial and viral infections.

Where Can You Get It?

Licorice is harvested from the plants' roots and underground stems. Licorice supplements are available as capsules, tablets and liquid extracts. It's available at most drugstores.

How Much Is Enough?

Because the research isn't clear, follow dosing instructions on the label.

Any Concerns?

Megadoses or long-term use can cause high blood pressure and deplete the body's potassium levels, which could lead to both heart and muscle problems. Pregnant women should avoid using licorice root as a supplement entirely.

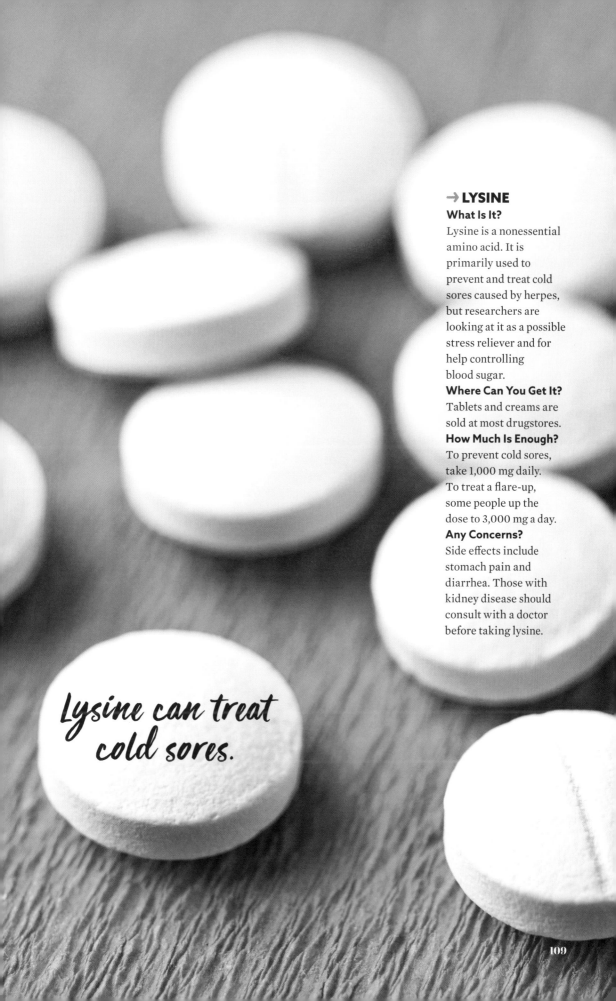

→ LYSINE

What Is It?
Lysine is a nonessential amino acid. It is primarily used to prevent and treat cold sores caused by herpes, but researchers are looking at it as a possible stress reliever and for help controlling blood sugar.

Where Can You Get It?
Tablets and creams are sold at most drugstores.

How Much Is Enough?
To prevent cold sores, take 1,000 mg daily. To treat a flare-up, some people up the dose to 3,000 mg a day.

Any Concerns?
Side effects include stomach pain and diarrhea. Those with kidney disease should consult with a doctor before taking lysine.

Lysine can treat cold sores.

M

→ MAGNESIUM

What Is It?

This mineral is essential for bones. Magnesium is also required for proper functioning of nerves, muscles and many other parts of the body. In the stomach, magnesium helps neutralize acid and move stools through the intestine. It can also be used to treat an irregular heartbeat.

Eat a healthy and complete diet— including plenty of spinach—and you should get enough magnesium.

Where Can You Get It?

Spinach, tofu, almonds, black beans, avocados and dark chocolate are just some of the food sources. People may need supplements, which are available in most drugstores.

How Much Is Enough?

The adult RDA is 400 to 420 mg for men and 310 to 320 mg for women.

Any Concerns?

Do not exceed the RDA. If the mineral builds up, it can trigger irregular heartbeat, low blood pressure, confusion, slowed breathing, coma or even death.

→ MANGANESE

What Is It?

An essential nutrient, manganese helps process cholesterol, carbohydrates and protein—it's involved in hundreds of key body processes. Researchers also believe it may play a key—and overlooked— role in bone formation. However, there is only minimal evidence that taking higher doses of this nutrient is necessary: You only need to make sure you're not deficient.

Where Can You Get It?

Manganese is found in several foods, including nuts, legumes, seeds, tea, whole grains and leafy green vegetables. It can also be made into supplements.

How Much Is Enough?

To meet the adult adequate intake, men need 2.3 mg; women need 1.8 mg.

Any Concerns?

Do not exceed more than 11 mg per day of manganese, especially if you are pregnant. It may also do harm to people with long-term liver disease.

Take note: Foods high in oxalic acid, such as sweet potatoes, can block manganese.

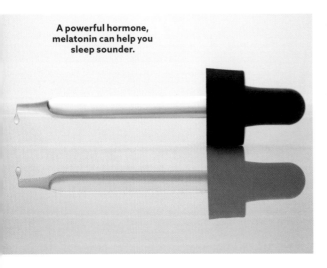

A powerful hormone, melatonin can help you sleep sounder.

→ MELATONIN

What Is It?

Found naturally in the body, melatonin's main job is to regulate your sleep-wake cycle. For people who have trouble sleeping or who battle insomnia, melatonin supplements may help.

Where Can You Get It?

It's sold as a supplement or drops that can be placed under the tongue.

How Much Is Enough?

Between 0.3 to 5 mg per day is considered safe.

Any Concerns?

Long-term use may cause headaches, depression, daytime sleepiness, dizziness, stomach cramps and irritability. You should not drive or use machinery for four to five hours after taking melatonin.

When milk thistle leaves are broken, a milky white substance comes out.

→ MILK THISTLE

What Is It?

The use of the milk thistle plant in a medicinal way dates back more than 2,000 years. It has been employed as a treatment for liver disorders, such as alcoholic hepatitis and cirrhosis; gallbladder problems; seasonal allergies; and heartburn. Researchers have found that it may also be effective in boosting the immune system. Studies have also shown that silymarin, a substance in milk thistle, may have an anti-cancer effect, both preventing the division of cancer cells and promoting cancer-cell death (apoptosis).

Where Can You Get It?

Available as capsules, powders and extracts in most drugstores.

How Much Is Enough?

Follow label instructions.

Any Concerns?

Milk thistle can act like a laxative. Some people may also experience nausea, diarrhea, indigestion and bloating.

N

→ NIACIN (VITAMIN B3)

What Is It?

This vitamin guides fats and sugars into cells, helping keep the body healthy. It can help lower cholesterol, and it may be effective in reducing atherosclerosis (hardening of the arteries). People also take it to treat Alzheimer's disease and erectile dysfunction, but evidence doesn't warrant these uses.

Where Can You Get It?

Vitamin B3 is found in foods such as yeast, meat, fish, milk, eggs, green vegetables and cereal grains. When taken as a supplement, niacin is often found in combination with other B vitamins.

How Much Is Enough?

For high cholesterol, between 50 mg and 12 grams a day, depending on the patient's condition. The adult RDA is 16 mg for men and 14 mg for women.

Any Concerns?

Do not take B3 if you have allergies, Crohn's disease, diabetes, gallbladder disease, gout, kidney disease, liver disease, ulcers, low blood pressure or thyroid disorders. Be aware that high doses can cause red, warm and itchy skin (aka the niacin flush).

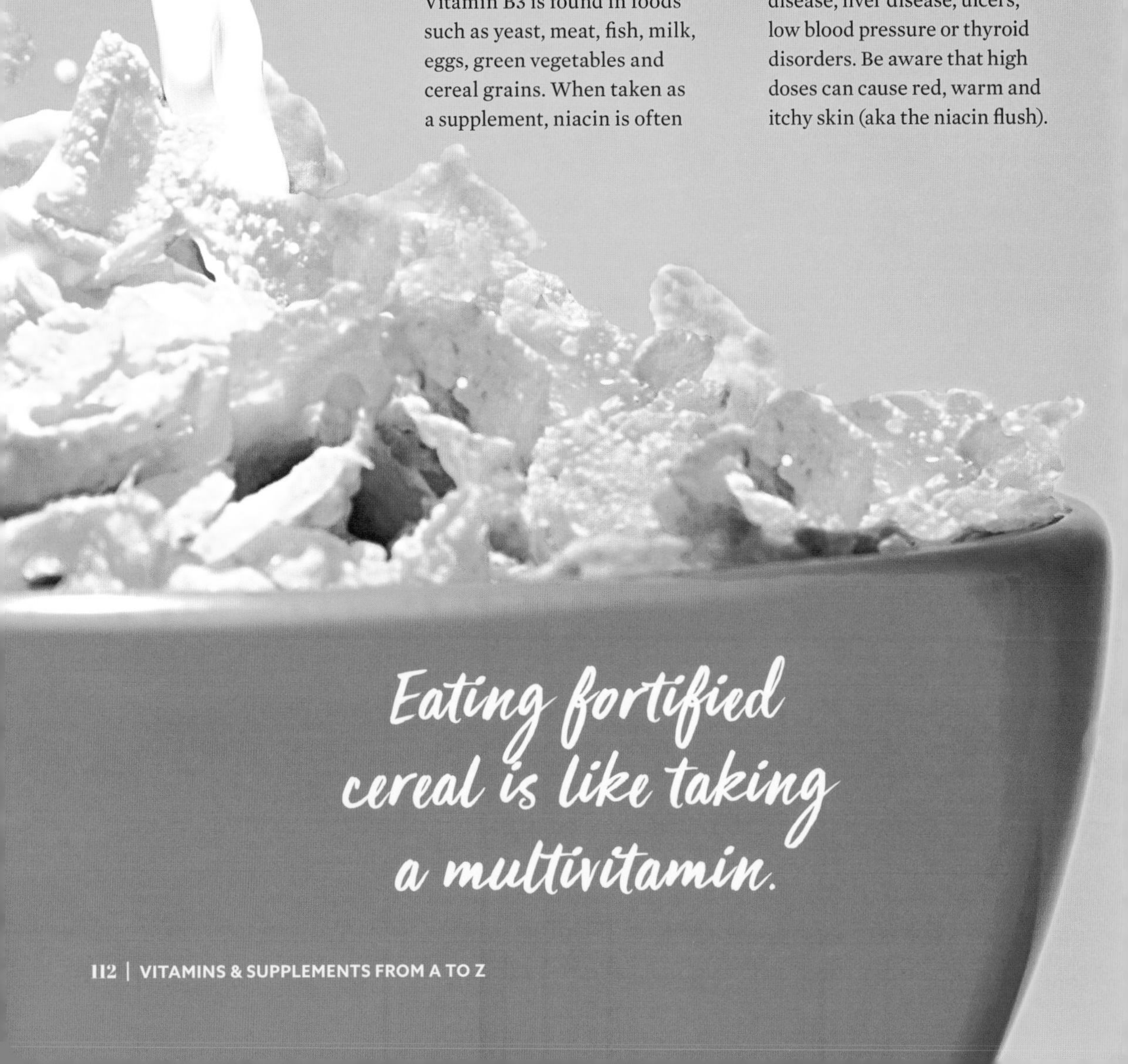

Eating fortified cereal is like taking a multivitamin.

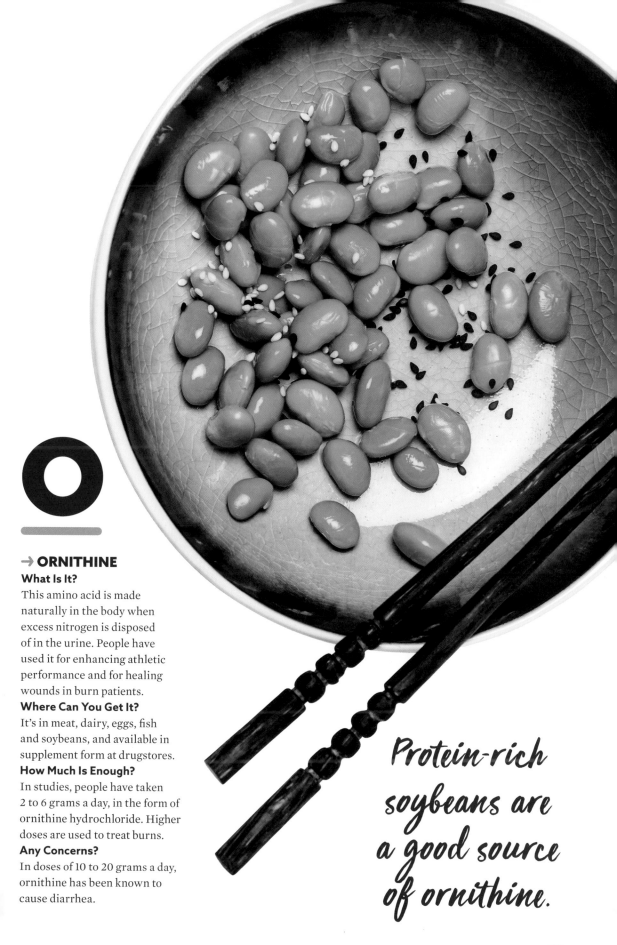

→ ORNITHINE

What Is It?

This amino acid is made naturally in the body when excess nitrogen is disposed of in the urine. People have used it for enhancing athletic performance and for healing wounds in burn patients.

Where Can You Get It?

It's in meat, dairy, eggs, fish and soybeans, and available in supplement form at drugstores.

How Much Is Enough?

In studies, people have taken 2 to 6 grams a day, in the form of ornithine hydrochloride. Higher doses are used to treat burns.

Any Concerns?

In doses of 10 to 20 grams a day, ornithine has been known to cause diarrhea.

Protein-rich soybeans are a good source of ornithine.

P

→ PANTOTHENIC ACID (VITAMIN B5)

What Is It?

People take it to treat conditions including acne, alcoholism, allergies, baldness, asthma and ADHD, but there is not enough scientific evidence to support this. B5 is an essential vitamin, helping the body process carbs, proteins and fats.

Where Can You Get It?

It's found in plants and animals, including meat, vegetables, cereal grains, legumes, eggs and milk. It is also available as a supplement.

How Much Is Enough?

Anywhere from 5 to 10 mg per day is usually enough to help prevent a deficiency and to help keep your body healthy.

Any Concerns?

Pregnant or breastfeeding women should not exceed more than 7 mg per day.

Almost all plant- and animal-based foods contain some pantothenic acid.

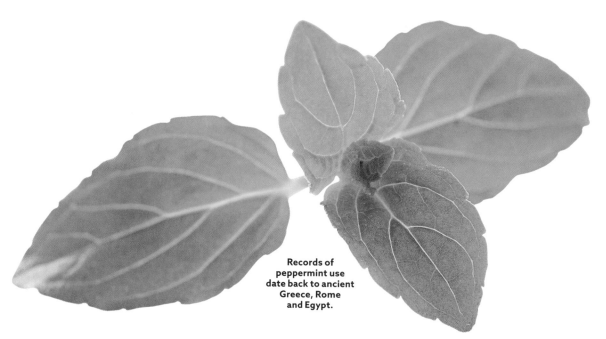

Records of peppermint use date back to ancient Greece, Rome and Egypt.

→ PEPPERMINT

What Is It?

The plant is used as a dietary supplement for irritable bowel syndrome (IBS), colds, headaches and many other common conditions. Peppermint oil is sometimes applied to the skin to help with headaches, muscle aches, itching and other problems. So far, research has only verified its effectiveness for IBS.

Where Can You Get It?

The leaf is available in teas, in capsules and as a liquid extract. Peppermint oil can be found in liquid solutions and capsules—including enteric-coated capsules.

How Much Is Enough?

The dosage varies depending on your intended usage. Follow the label directions or check with your doctor.

Any Concerns?

Excessive doses of peppermint oil can be toxic. Side effects can include allergic reactions and heartburn.

→ PHENYLALANINE

What Is It?

An amino acid, it comes in three forms: D-phenylalanine (made in a laboratory), L-phenylalanine (the natural form found in proteins) and a synthesized laboratory mix called DL-phenylalanine. D-phenylalanine may be useful in treating chronic pain and Parkinson's disease. L-phenylalanine has been shown to be useful in the treatment of vitiligo—a condition in which pigment is lost from the skin, resulting in white patches.

Where Can You Get It?

L-phenylalanine can be found in meat, fish, eggs, cheese and milk. D-phenylalanine is only available in supplement form.

How Much Is Enough?

Follow the dosing instructions on the label.

Any Concerns?

L-phenylalanine is generally safe when consumed in amounts found in food. There is not enough information on the safety of D-phenylalanine.

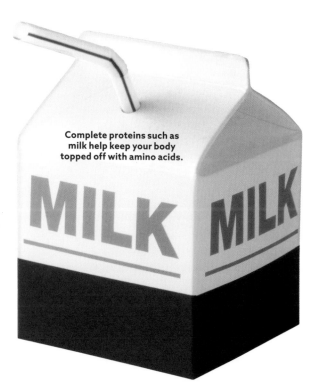

Complete proteins such as milk help keep your body topped off with amino acids.

MILK MILK

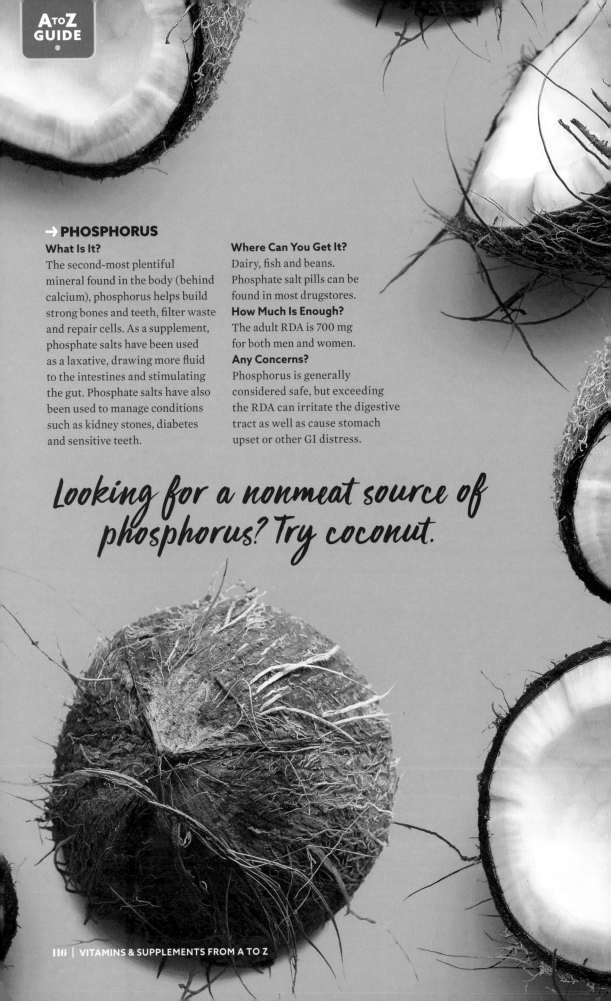

→ PHOSPHORUS

What Is It?

The second-most plentiful mineral found in the body (behind calcium), phosphorus helps build strong bones and teeth, filter waste and repair cells. As a supplement, phosphate salts have been used as a laxative, drawing more fluid to the intestines and stimulating the gut. Phosphate salts have also been used to manage conditions such as kidney stones, diabetes and sensitive teeth.

Where Can You Get It?

Dairy, fish and beans. Phosphate salt pills can be found in most drugstores.

How Much Is Enough?

The adult RDA is 700 mg for both men and women.

Any Concerns?

Phosphorus is generally considered safe, but exceeding the RDA can irritate the digestive tract as well as cause stomach upset or other GI distress.

Looking for a nonmeat source of phosphorus? Try coconut.

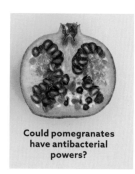

Could pomegranates have antibacterial powers?

→ POMEGRANATE

What Is It?
Researchers have long studied pomegranate. A recent study of about 100 dialysis patients suggested that pomegranate juice may help ward off infections. In the study, the patients who were given pomegranate juice three times a week for a year had fewer hospitalizations for infections and fewer signs of inflammation.

Where Can You Get It?
In addition to the fruit, you can get pomegranate in capsules, extracts, teas, powders and juices, sold in most drugstores.

How Much Is Enough?
Follow the label instructions.

Any Concerns?
Some people, particularly those with plant allergies, should use caution when taking pomegranate-related products.

→ POTASSIUM

What Is It?
This essential mineral helps the brain communicate with the rest of the body by facilitating nerve transmissions. It also helps to maintain fluid balance and may help lower blood pressure and reduce the risk of stroke.

Where Can You Get It?
Food sources of potassium include fruits (especially dried fruits), cereals, beans, milk and vegetables. It can also be made into supplements, sold at most drugstores.

How Much Is Enough?
The normal adult daily requirement is 4.7 grams.

Any Concerns?
Too much can be extremely dangerous and can cause feelings of burning or tingling, generalized weakness, paralysis, listlessness and dizziness.

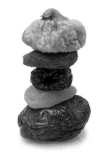

You can get a concentrated dose of potassium from dried fruits.

→ PYRIDOXINE (VITAMIN B6)

What Is It?
Vitamin B6 is an essential vitamin that helps the body make neurotransmitters that carry information between cells. It also plays a vital role in the growth and development of the brain, nerves, skin and other parts of the body. Researchers have tested it in patients with blood vessel disease, high cholesterol and elevated blood pressure.

Where Can You Get It?
B6 can be found in certain foods, such as cereals, beans, vegetables, liver, meat and eggs. It can also be made in a lab.

How Much Is Enough?
The adult RDA is 1.3 to 1.7 mg for men and 1.3 to 1.5 mg for women.

Any Concerns?
Exceeding the RDA can cause nausea, vomiting, stomach pain and headaches. Avoid taking B6 if you have diabetes, as it can increase your risk of certain cancers. And don't mix B6 with blood pressure medications.

The B6 you get from meat can help treat anemia—just like iron does.

→ PYRUVATE

What Is It?
The body produces the antioxidant pyruvate when it breaks down sugar (glucose). Pyruvic acid seems to help the outer layer of skin cells slough off, which accounts for its use in reversing aging due to sun exposure.

Where Can You Get It?
There are small amounts in red apples, cheese, dark beer and red wine. Pyruvate can be made into supplements that are sold at most drugstores.

How Much Is Enough?
People have used a 50% pyruvic acid peel, applied once weekly for four weeks, for aging skin.

Any Concerns?
Supplements may worsen existing diarrhea and irritable bowel syndrome. Applying too much pyruvate acid peel can cause severe skin burning; use it only with a dermatologist's supervision. The peel should only be applied to small patches of skin.

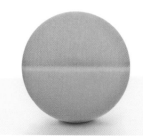

Pyruvate can help with weight loss by increasing the breakdown of fat in the body.

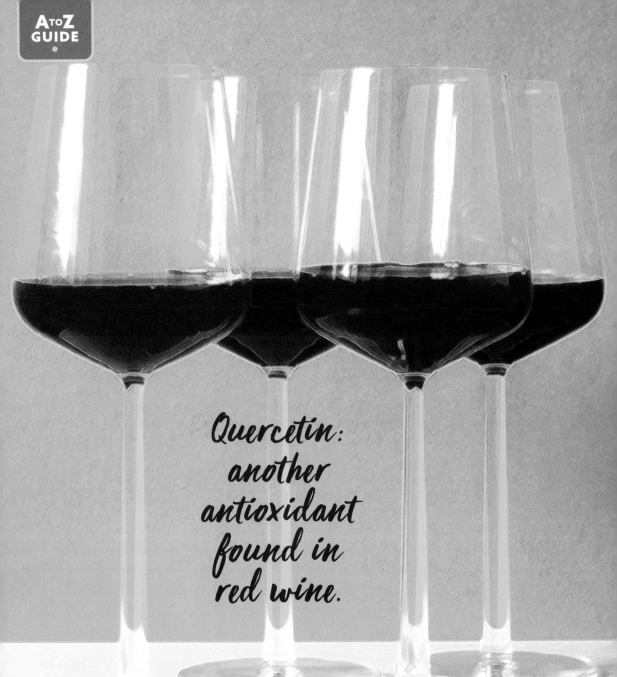

Quercetin: another antioxidant found in red wine.

→ QUERCETIN

What Is It?

Quercetin is a plant pigment that is found in red wine, onions, green tea, apples, berries and some herbs. Scientist believe it has antioxidant effects that can help reduce prostate inflammation; it also shows promise for treating atherosclerosis, high cholesterol, heart disease and some circulation issues.

Where Can You Get It?

In food and supplements.

How Much Is Enough?

Doctors recommend 500 mg of quercetin, taken twice daily, for prostate pain.

Any Concerns?

Effects of long-term use are not known. It may cause headaches and tingling of limbs; very high doses may damage the kidneys.

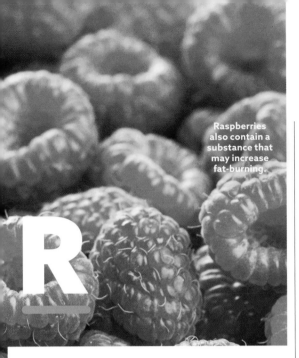

Raspberries also contain a substance that may increase fat-burning.

R

→ RED CLOVER

What Is It?

This plant originates in Europe and Asia, although it's now grown all over the world. Red clover is a good source of isoflavones, a type of antioxidant. The body converts isoflavones to phytoestrogen, an estrogen-like substance. When researchers have tested it in women, red clover seemed to help raise levels of good cholesterol, ease symptoms of menopause and boost bone growth, although more research needs to be done to verify the results.

Where Can You Get It?

Red clover is made into teas, tinctures, pills, powders, oils and extracts that are sold at many drugstores.

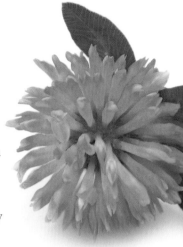

Red clover is used as a flavoring in some foods.

How Much Is Enough?

Depending on the use, the dosage can vary. Follow the label instructions or get advice from a medical professional.

Any Concerns?

In some women, red clover can cause side effects such as a rash, muscle aches, headache, nausea and vaginal bleeding (spotting).

→ RASPBERRY KETONE

What Is It?

A chemical that comes from red raspberries, raspberry ketone is used to boost metabolism and increase weight loss. It may assist hormones that reduce appetite as well, although more evidence is needed for this use.

Where Can You Get It?

It's in raspberries, of course, but also in kiwi, peaches, grapes, apples and other berries.

How Much Is Enough?

Follow label instructions.

Any Concerns?

It may cause nervousness and rapid heartbeat.

→ RIBOFLAVIN (B2)

What Is It?

Your body needs this water-soluble B vitamin to keep your skin, digestive tract and blood cells healthy. You also depend upon it to process other B vitamins, and together, they're critical for metabolizing the energy your body runs on.

Where Can You Get It?

Milk, meat, eggs, nuts, enriched flour and green vegetables. It is also available in pill form.

How Much Is Enough?

The adult daily RDA for men is 1.3 mg; for women, it's 1.1 mg.

Any Concerns?

Exceeding the RDA of vitamin B2 might cause side effects such as diarrhea, migraines, an increase in urine output and other symptoms. Pregnant women should not take more than 1.4 mg a day, and breastfeeding women should not take more than 1.6 mg a day.

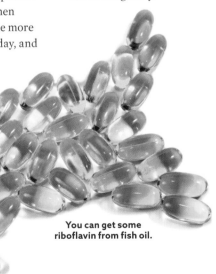

You can get some riboflavin from fish oil.

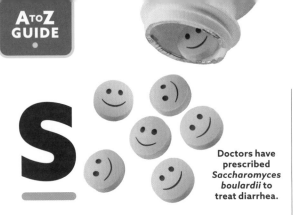

Doctors have prescribed *Saccharomyces boulardii* to treat diarrhea.

→ SACCHAROMYCES BOULARDII

What Is It?

This probiotic is actually a yeast. Like other probiotics, it's known for helping protect against gut issues; however, it can also ease acne, yeast infections and, potentially, Lyme disease.

Where Can You Get It?

It can be made into supplements and is sold at most drugstores.

How Much Is Enough?

There is no RDA for this probiotic, but health professionals usually recommend anywhere from 250 mg to 1 gram a day.

Any Concerns?

It is overall safe to take orally for up to 15 months, though it may cause an increase in flatulence. In rare instances, the supplement might lead to serious fungal infections that spread throughout the body.

→ SAGE

What Is It?

The plant is used as a dietary supplement for digestive issues, sore mouth or throat, memory loss and depression. It may also help boost memory and speed learning.

Where Can You Get It?

Sage leaves or their extracts are available as liquids, throat sprays, tablets, lozenges and capsules.

How Much Is Enough?

In some studies, people took 1 gram of sage per day.

Any Concerns?

If used over long periods of time, the leaves and oil of sage may trigger side effects such as nervousness, dizziness, rapid heart rate, seizures and even kidney damage.

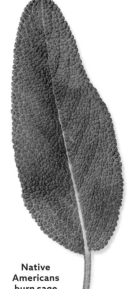

Native Americans burn sage to promote healing, wisdom and longevity.

→ SAMe

What Is It?

The body forms this molecule as a building block for other substances that help ease pain, relieve depression and ward off liver disease. People who don't make enough SAMe naturally may be helped by taking SAMe as a supplement.

Where Can You Get It?

A synthetic version of SAMe is available in supplement form in most drugstores.

How Much Is Enough?

Depending on the condition, SAMe dosages range from 600–1,600 mg.

Any Concerns?

SAMe is generally safe when taken by mouth, given intravenously or when injected as a shot, appropriately. For some patients, the supplement can sometimes cause gas, vomiting, diarrhea, constipation, dry mouth, headache, mild insomnia, anorexia, sweating, dizziness and nervousness; this is especially true when taken at higher doses. It can also make some people with depression feel anxious.

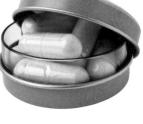

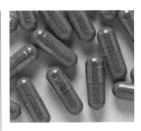

Saw palmetto may slow the growth of tumor cells, say researchers.

→ SAW PALMETTO

What Is It?

The fruit of this palm-like plant is used in an extract to treat symptoms of an enlarged prostate (benign prostatic hyperplasia, or BPH). People have also taken it to boost libido and increase fertility. It may also have anti-inflammatory properties.

Where Can You Get It?

The berries are dried and sold whole or ground up and placed in capsules or tablets; extracts of the fruit are used in tinctures and teas.

How Much Is Enough?

For an enlarged prostate, doctors recommend a dosage of 160 mg, two times a day, to decrease symptoms.

Any Concerns?

Research shows saw palmetto is well tolerated by most people. Mild side effects may include digestive symptoms, dizziness and headache. In rare instances, it has caused liver damage. Only take it under a doctor's supervision.

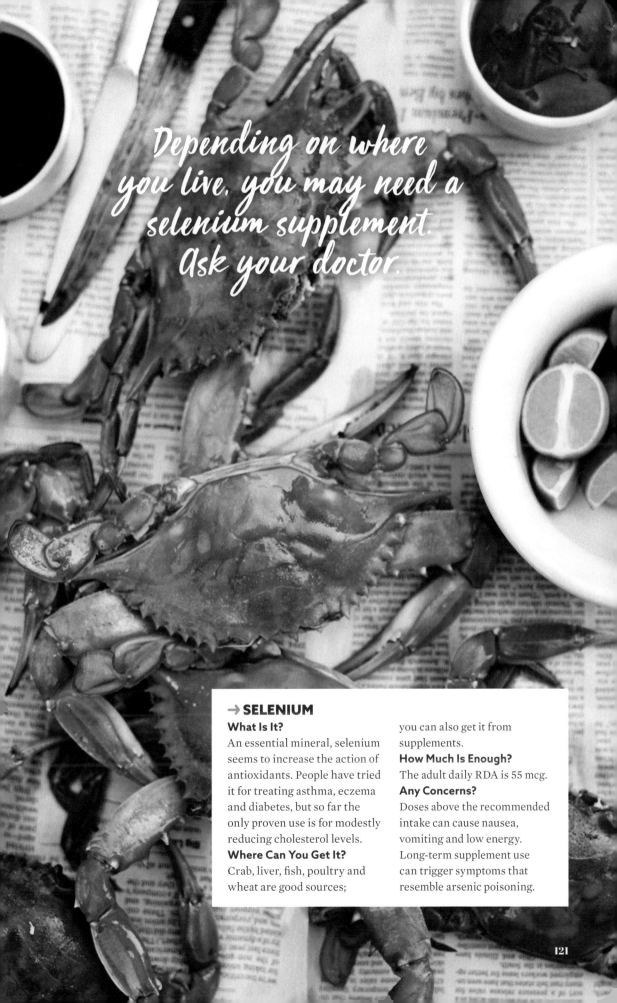

Depending on where you live, you may need a selenium supplement. Ask your doctor.

→ SELENIUM

What Is It?

An essential mineral, selenium seems to increase the action of antioxidants. People have tried it for treating asthma, eczema and diabetes, but so far the only proven use is for modestly reducing cholesterol levels.

Where Can You Get It?

Crab, liver, fish, poultry and wheat are good sources; you can also get it from supplements.

How Much Is Enough?

The adult daily RDA is 55 mcg.

Any Concerns?

Doses above the recommended intake can cause nausea, vomiting and low energy. Long-term supplement use can trigger symptoms that resemble arsenic poisoning.

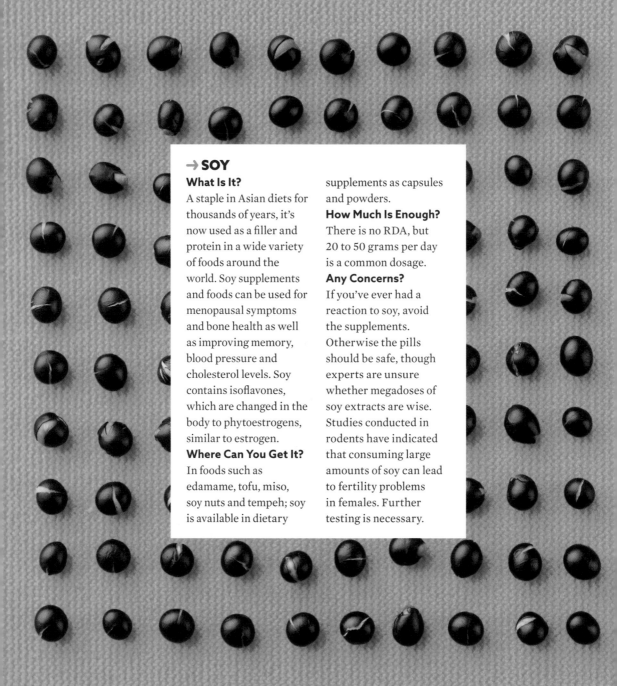

→ SOY

What Is It?

A staple in Asian diets for thousands of years, it's now used as a filler and protein in a wide variety of foods around the world. Soy supplements and foods can be used for menopausal symptoms and bone health as well as improving memory, blood pressure and cholesterol levels. Soy contains isoflavones, which are changed in the body to phytoestrogens, similar to estrogen.

Where Can You Get It?

In foods such as edamame, tofu, miso, soy nuts and tempeh; soy is available in dietary supplements as capsules and powders.

How Much Is Enough?

There is no RDA, but 20 to 50 grams per day is a common dosage.

Any Concerns?

If you've ever had a reaction to soy, avoid the supplements. Otherwise the pills should be safe, though experts are unsure whether megadoses of soy extracts are wise. Studies conducted in rodents have indicated that consuming large amounts of soy can lead to fertility problems in females. Further testing is necessary.

You can eat soybeans in a variety of ways: cooked, as part of tofu or dry-roasted.

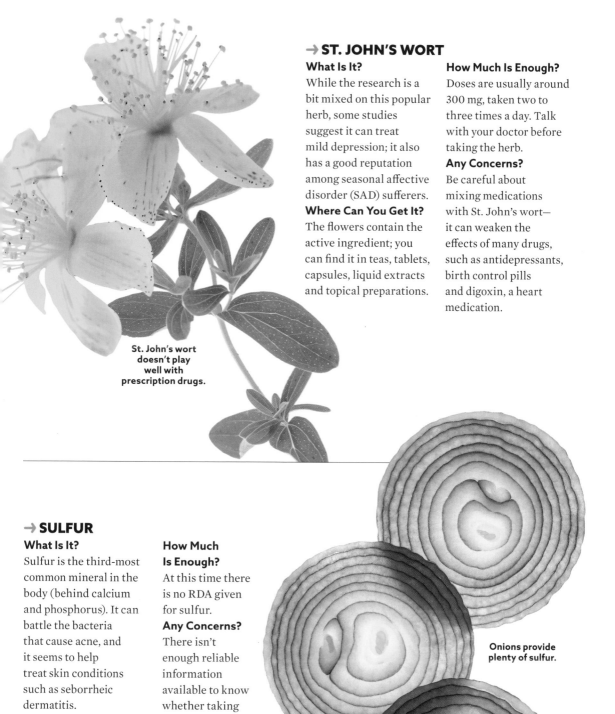

→ ST. JOHN'S WORT

What Is It?
While the research is a bit mixed on this popular herb, some studies suggest it can treat mild depression; it also has a good reputation among seasonal affective disorder (SAD) sufferers.

Where Can You Get It?
The flowers contain the active ingredient; you can find it in teas, tablets, capsules, liquid extracts and topical preparations.

How Much Is Enough?
Doses are usually around 300 mg, taken two to three times a day. Talk with your doctor before taking the herb.

Any Concerns?
Be careful about mixing medications with St. John's wort—it can weaken the effects of many drugs, such as antidepressants, birth control pills and digoxin, a heart medication.

St. John's wort doesn't play well with prescription drugs.

→ SULFUR

What Is It?
Sulfur is the third-most common mineral in the body (behind calcium and phosphorus). It can battle the bacteria that cause acne, and it seems to help treat skin conditions such as seborrheic dermatitis.

Where Can You Get It?
Sulfur is found in garlic, onions and broccoli, cabbage and other sulfuric foods. It's also available in supplements.

How Much Is Enough?
At this time there is no RDA given for sulfur.

Any Concerns?
There isn't enough reliable information available to know whether taking sulfur as an oral medication is safe, although minimal findings suggest that doing so might cause diarrhea.

Onions provide plenty of sulfur.

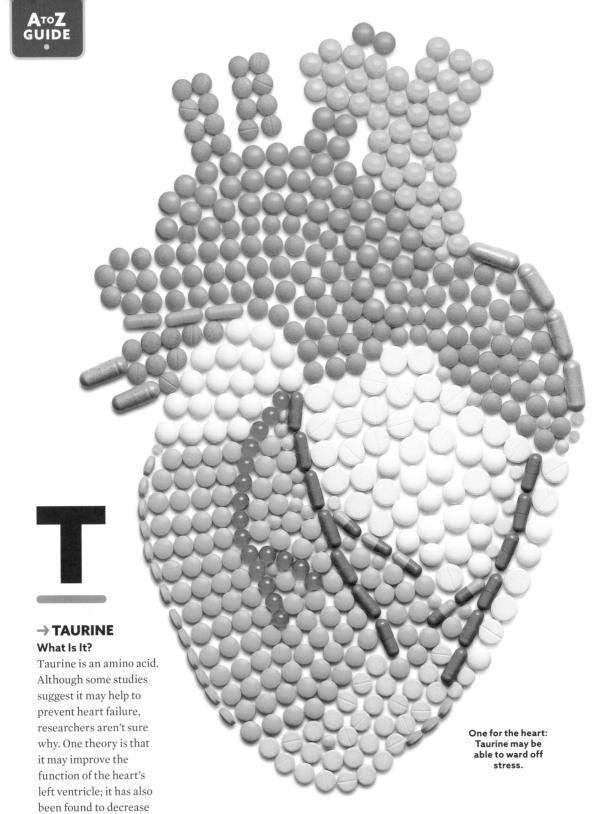

One for the heart: Taurine may be able to ward off stress.

T

→ TAURINE

What Is It?

Taurine is an amino acid. Although some studies suggest it may help to prevent heart failure, researchers aren't sure why. One theory is that it may improve the function of the heart's left ventricle; it has also been found to decrease blood pressure and ease the effects of stress on the entire nervous system.

Where Can You Get It?

The best food sources are meat and fish; it's also in pills.

How Much Is Enough?

From 2 to 6 grams per day have been used for congestive heart failure.

Any Concerns?

No side effects are reported for taurine taken orally at the proper dosage. Discuss it with your doctor.

→ THIAMINE (B1)

What Is It?

You need it to burn carbs, and it can treat metabolic and brain disorders if you happen to be low in B vitamins. Interestingly, vitamin B1 may help protect against cataracts; kidney disease, in people with diabetes; and painful menstruation.

Where Can You Get It?

Foods such as yeast, cereal grains, beans, nuts and meat; you can also get it in supplements.

How Much Is Enough?

As a dietary supplement, adults commonly use 1–2 mg per day, according to research. For adults looking to reduce the risk of cataracts, a 10 mg daily dosage is recommended. Pregnant and breastfeeding women should not exceed 1.5 mg per day.

Any Concerns?

It's safe for pregnant and breast-feeding women at the recommended dosage. However, not enough is known about exceeding the recommended amount. People who have liver problems, and heavy drinkers, may not be able to absorb enough and need to get more.

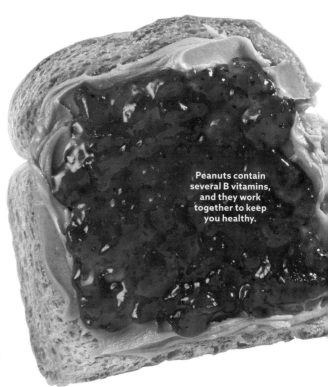

Peanuts contain several B vitamins, and they work together to keep you healthy.

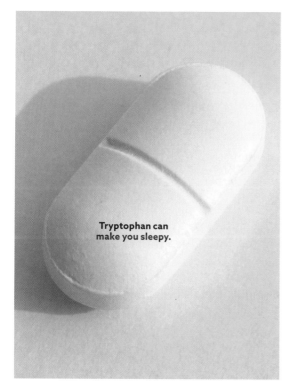

Tryptophan can make you sleepy.

→ TRYPTOPHAN

What Is It?

This essential amino acid is converted to serotonin, a hormone tied to mood. Tryptophan supplements can be effective for insomnia, sleep apnea, depression and anxiety.

Where Can You Get It?

Tryptophan naturally comes from most plants and animals—and in supplements.

How Much Is Enough?

Follow the label instructions and consult a medical professional before taking.

Any Concerns?

In 1990, tryptophan supplements were recalled from the market because of some safety concerns. After the problem was traced back to a single manufacturer in Japan, the supplements remained embargoed until 2007, when they came back on the market. Possible side effects include heartburn; stomach pain; belching and gas; nausea; vomiting; diarrhea; and loss of appetite. It can also cause headache, light-headedness, drowsiness, dry mouth, visual blurring, muscle weakness and some sexual problems.

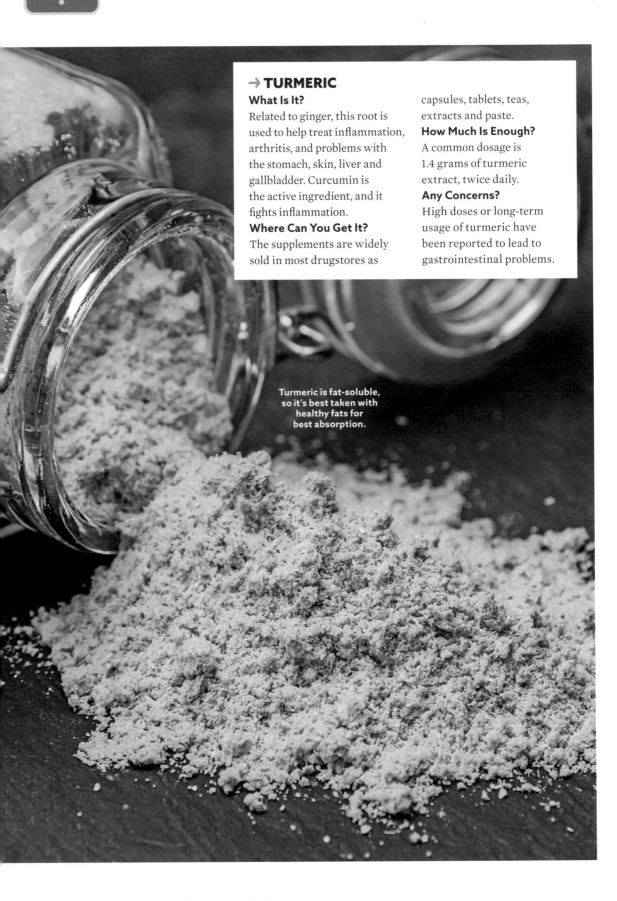

→ TURMERIC

What Is It?

Related to ginger, this root is used to help treat inflammation, arthritis, and problems with the stomach, skin, liver and gallbladder. Curcumin is the active ingredient, and it fights inflammation.

Where Can You Get It?

The supplements are widely sold in most drugstores as capsules, tablets, teas, extracts and paste.

How Much Is Enough?

A common dosage is 1.4 grams of turmeric extract, twice daily.

Any Concerns?

High doses or long-term usage of turmeric have been reported to lead to gastrointestinal problems.

Turmeric is fat-soluble, so it's best taken with healthy fats for best absorption.

→ TYROSINE

What Is It?

Another essential amino acid: The body uses tyrosine to make neurotransmitters. People mainly take tyrosine for mental alertness and better memory. It is also used for depression and ADHD, though evidence for effectiveness to treat these conditions is mixed.

Where Can You Get It?

From complete protein foods such as meat, poultry, dairy, nuts and seeds. Tyrosine can be made into supplements, and is sold at most drugstores.

How Much Is Enough?

There is no RDA, but 150 mg a day, in split doses, has been used to improve alertness in those suffering from a lack of sleep.

Any Concerns?

Tyrosine is considered safe, but some people have reported side effects that include nausea, headache, fatigue, heartburn and joint pain.

Tyrosine improves learning, memory and alertness, especially under stress.

U

→ UMCKALOABO

What Is It?

A flowering plant that is found in South Africa, umckaloabo (aka South African geranium) is often used to treat upper respiratory infections. Researchers think that it might work by killing bacteria. It is mainly used for a variety of respiratory ailments, including bronchitis, sinusitis, sore throat, tonsillitis and the common cold.

Where Can You Get It?

This plant can be made into supplements, which are sold at most drugstores.

How Much Is Enough?

Doctors recommend 10 to 30 mg, three times a day, for bronchitis.

Any Concerns?

It's considered generally safe, but there is not enough information to know if it is safe when taken for longer periods of time.

Get some flower power.

V

→ VALERIAN

What Is It?

People use this herb for neurological conditions such as anxiety, insomnia, depression, and symptoms of menopause, such as hot flashes.

Where Can You Get It?

In capsules, tablets, liquid extracts and teas.

How Much Is Enough?

For sleep problems, 400 to 900 mg of valerian extract up to two hours before bed.

Any Concerns?

Valerian is considered safe, although a few side effects have been reported, including headache, dizziness, confusion, itching and digestive disturbances.

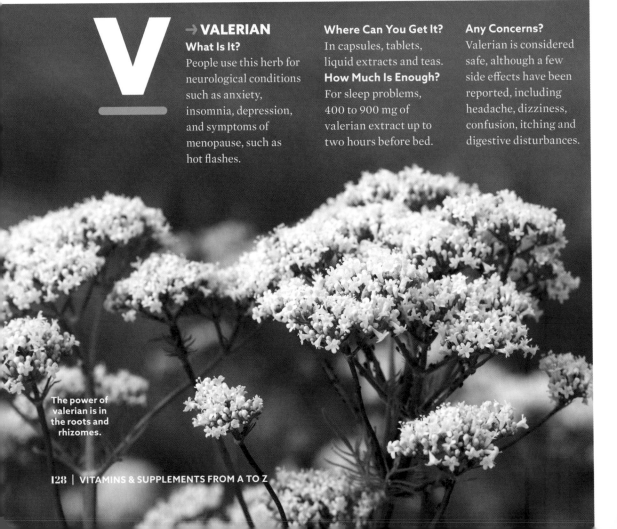

The power of valerian is in the roots and rhizomes.

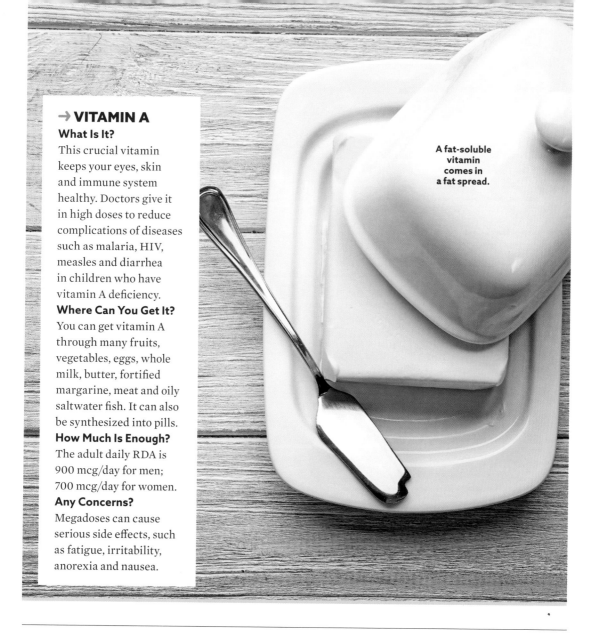

→ VITAMIN A
What Is It?
This crucial vitamin keeps your eyes, skin and immune system healthy. Doctors give it in high doses to reduce complications of diseases such as malaria, HIV, measles and diarrhea in children who have vitamin A deficiency.

Where Can You Get It?
You can get vitamin A through many fruits, vegetables, eggs, whole milk, butter, fortified margarine, meat and oily saltwater fish. It can also be synthesized into pills.

How Much Is Enough?
The adult daily RDA is 900 mcg/day for men; 700 mcg/day for women.

Any Concerns?
Megadoses can cause serious side effects, such as fatigue, irritability, anorexia and nausea.

A fat-soluble vitamin comes in a fat spread.

→ VITAMIN B12
What Is It?
This is an essential vitamin—your body needs it to keep your brain, nerves, blood cells and other crucial organs working properly. It can help reduce levels of homocysteine in the blood—a risk factor for heart disease—and may help prevent age-related macular degeneration (a leading cause of blindness) and nerve damage from shingles.

Where Can You Get It?
Look for it in foods such as meat, fish and dairy products; you can also get it in supplements.

How Much Is Enough?
The adult daily RDA is 1.8 mcg. After 50, talk to your doctor about getting more.

Any Concerns?
Pregnant women should stick to the recommended dosage. Avoid taking B12 after postsurgical stent placement or if you have an allergy or sensitivity.

As we age, we absorb less B12; make sure to get plenty from your diet.

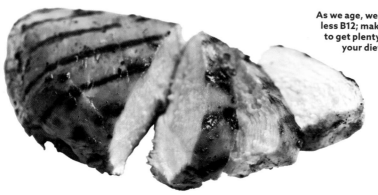

→ VITAMIN C

What Is It?

Maybe the most commonly known nutrient, vitamin C helps keep your immune system strong. As a supplement, it's most often taken to treat the common cold.

Where Can You Get It?

Most commonly found in citrus fruits, you can also get it from supplements.

How Much Is Enough?

The daily recommended dietary allowances (RDAs) are 90 mg for men and 75 mg for women. For treating or preventing the common cold, take 1 to 3 grams a day.

Any Concerns?

More than 2,000 mg a day raises the risk of severe diarrhea and kidney stones.

Citrus fruits are also packed with fiber and are good for the heart.

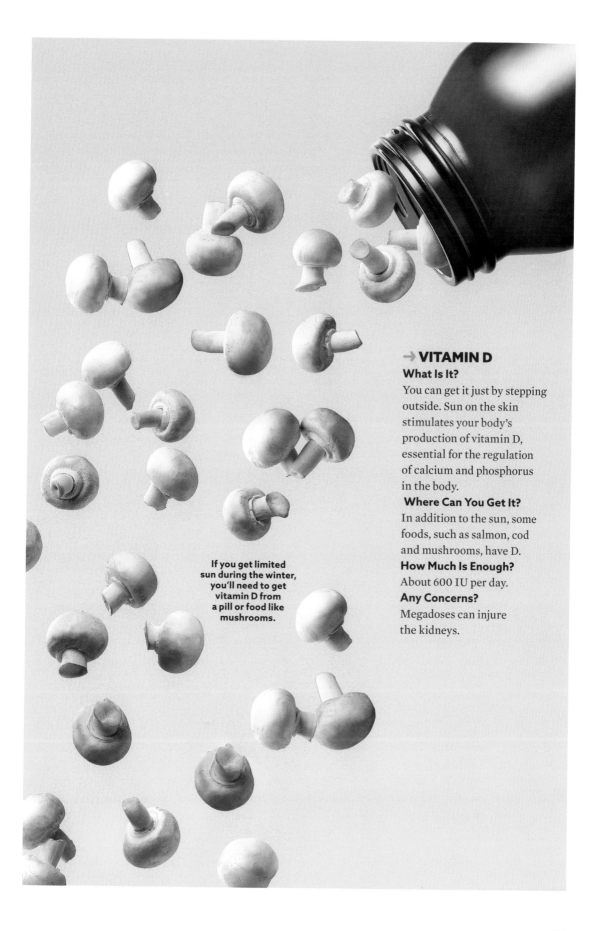

→ VITAMIN D

What Is It?

You can get it just by stepping outside. Sun on the skin stimulates your body's production of vitamin D, essential for the regulation of calcium and phosphorus in the body.

Where Can You Get It?

In addition to the sun, some foods, such as salmon, cod and mushrooms, have D.

How Much Is Enough?

About 600 IU per day.

Any Concerns?

Megadoses can injure the kidneys.

If you get limited sun during the winter, you'll need to get vitamin D from a pill or food like mushrooms.

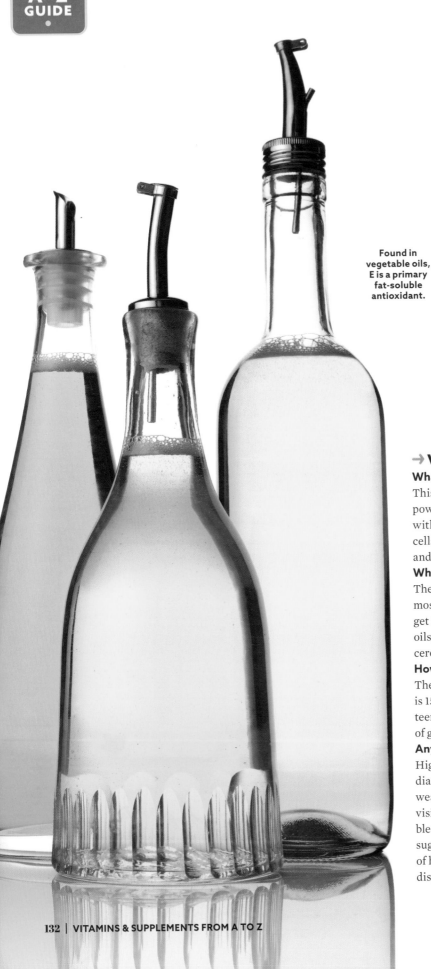

Found in
vegetable oils,
E is a primary
fat-soluble
antioxidant.

→ VITAMIN E

What Is It?

This essential vitamin, a powerful antioxidant, works with vitamin C to keep your cells and tissues healthy and safe from free radicals.

Where Can You Get It?

The supplements are available in most drugstores, but you can also get it from produce, plant-based oils, meat, eggs and breakfast cereals.

How Much Is Enough?

The recommended daily intake is 15 mg per day (or 22.5 IU) for teens and adults, regardless of gender.

Any Concerns?

High doses can cause nausea, diarrhea, stomach cramps, fatigue, weakness, headache, blurred vision, rash and bruising and bleeding. Although some studies suggest it could decrease the risk of heart attack, later research disproved this benefit.

→ VITAMIN K

What Is It?

This essential vitamin helps blood to form clots and bones to grow—calcium relies on it to strengthen your skeleton. Although there are several forms of vitamin K, the version called K1 is considered less toxic while offering more benefits. Researchers have tested K topically to treat bruises, scars, burns, stretch marks, and other skin conditions.

Where Can You Get It?

Available as a supplement, but you can find it naturally in leafy green vegetables, broccoli and Brussels sprouts.

How Much Is Enough?

For adults, the adequate intake for men is 120 mcg, and for women, 90 mcg.

Any Concerns?

The two forms of vitamin K (vitamin K1 and vitamin K2) are generally safe for most people when taken orally or injected, as is required for certain medical conditions. If you are on dialysis for kidney disease, an excess of vitamin K can be detrimental. Talk to your doctor if you are on blood thinners.

Vitamin K is essential in healing injuries—it helps blood clot and bones mend.

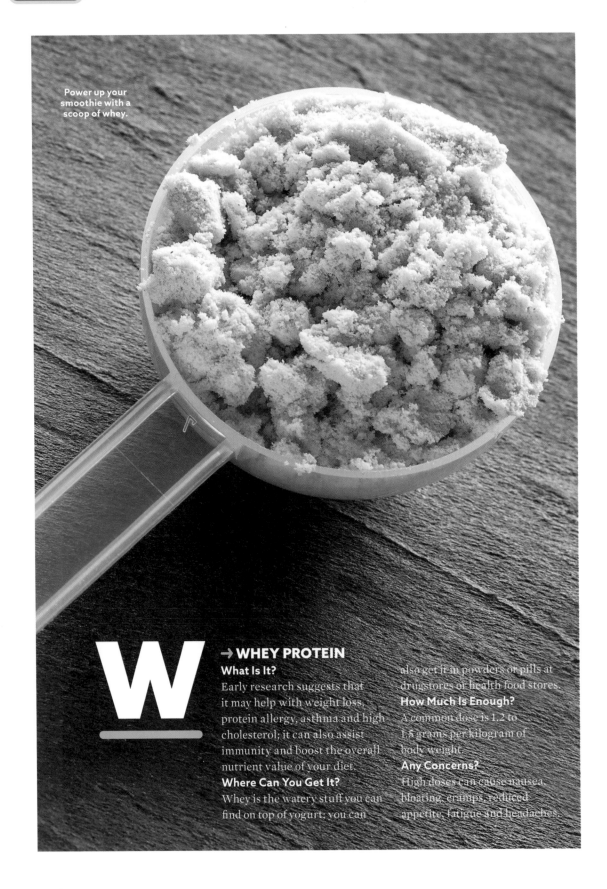

Power up your smoothie with a scoop of whey.

W

→ WHEY PROTEIN

What Is It?

Early research suggests that it may help with weight loss, protein allergy, asthma and high cholesterol; it can also assist immunity and boost the overall nutrient value of your diet.

Where Can You Get It?

Whey is the watery stuff you can find on top of yogurt; you can also get it in powders or pills at drugstores or health food stores.

How Much Is Enough?

A common dose is 1.2 to 1.5 grams per kilogram of body weight.

Any Concerns?

High doses can cause nausea, bloating, cramps, reduced appetite, fatigue and headaches.

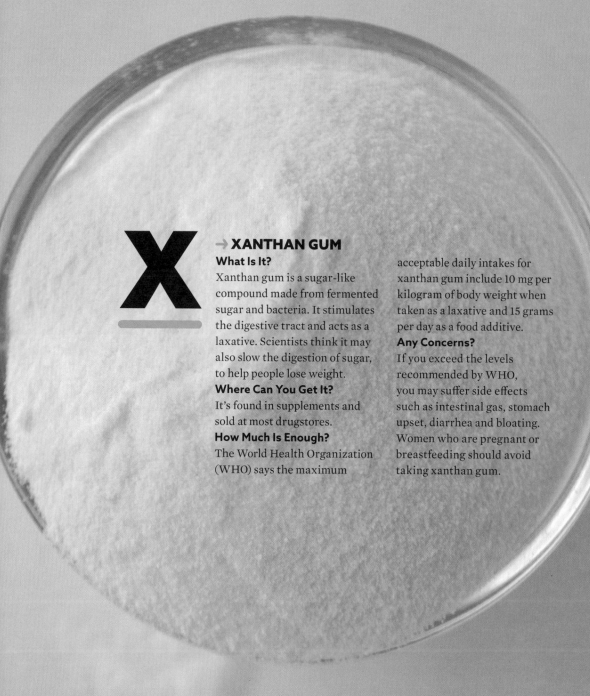

X

→XANTHAN GUM

What Is It?

Xanthan gum is a sugar-like compound made from fermented sugar and bacteria. It stimulates the digestive tract and acts as a laxative. Scientists think it may also slow the digestion of sugar, to help people lose weight.

Where Can You Get It?

It's found in supplements and sold at most drugstores.

How Much Is Enough?

The World Health Organization (WHO) says the maximum acceptable daily intakes for xanthan gum include 10 mg per kilogram of body weight when taken as a laxative and 15 grams per day as a food additive.

Any Concerns?

If you exceed the levels recommended by WHO, you may suffer side effects such as intestinal gas, stomach upset, diarrhea and bloating. Women who are pregnant or breastfeeding should avoid taking xanthan gum.

You can stay regular with xanthan gum supplements.

Y

→ YERBA MATE

What Is It?

This plant contains caffeine and other chemicals that stimulate the brain, the heart and the muscles lining blood vessels. It's used as a stimulant to counteract mental and physical fatigue and to treat chronic fatigue syndrome. People have tried it for heart-related issues including irregular heartbeat and low blood pressure, as well as for weight loss and better digestion.

Where Can You Get It?

As a tea or in supplements, sold at most drugstores.

How Much Is Enough?

More research is needed before experts can determine this plant's appropriate range of doses.

Any Concerns?

When taken in large amounts or for long periods of time, yerba mate may raise the risk of mouth, esophageal, laryngeal, kidney, bladder and lung cancers.

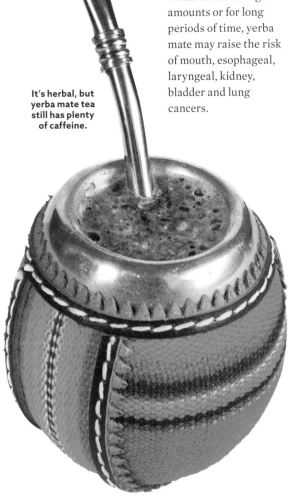

It's herbal, but yerba mate tea still has plenty of caffeine.

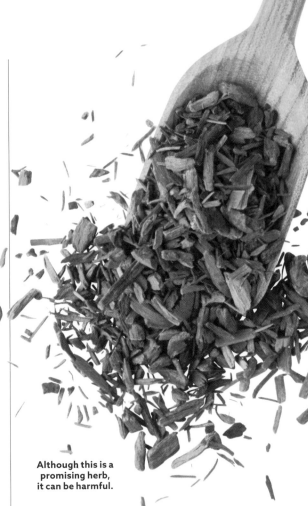

Although this is a promising herb, it can be harmful.

→ YOHIMBE

What Is It?

The bark of this African evergreen tree has been used by local tribes as a sexual stimulant. The active ingredient, yohimbine, seems to increase blood flow to the genitals, and people take it to boost libido, treat erectile dysfunction and address other sex issues in men and women. Researchers are studying whether it can help with depression, exhaustion, chest pain, weight loss and other medical problems, although the results aren't clear yet.

Where Can You Get It?

Yohimbine hydrochloride is available as a prescription drug for erectile dysfunction. This is different from dietary supplements made from the bark of the tree, which can be found in drugstores.

How Much Is Enough?

For problems with sexual performance, 15 to 30 mg daily.

Any Concerns?

Side effects can be dangerous and include seizures, high blood pressure and heart attacks. Take only under a doctor's supervision.

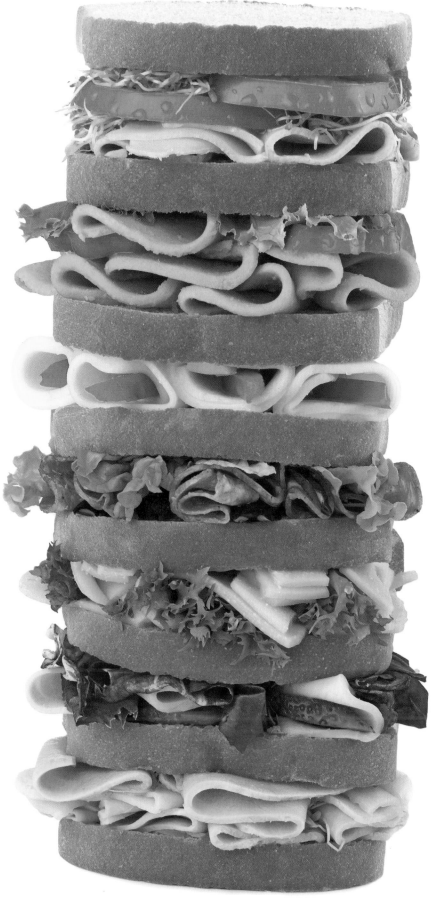

Z

ZINC

What Is It?
This mineral supports immunity and metabolism. People use oral zinc to help fight colds.

Where Can You Get It?
Food sources include chicken, red meat and fortified breakfast cereals; it's also in supplements.

How Much Is Enough?
The RDA is 8 mg for women; 11 mg for men.

Any Concerns?
Stick to the RDA to avoid side effects.

Call this one the Zinc Special: Meats, cereals and grains can provide all the zinc you need.

A

Acai berries, 76

Acetyl-L-carnitine, 72

Adequate intake (AI), 16–17

    biotin (vitamin B7), 81

    choline, 86

    chromium, 88

    manganese, 110

    vitamin K, 133

ADHD. *See* Attention-deficit
    hyperactivity/disorder
    (ADHD)

Adulteration, of supplements,
    27

Age/Aging

    anti-aging therapy and, 90

    mental stimulation activities
      and, 73

    normal symptoms of,
      malnutrition vs., 48

    nutrient deficiency and, 28

AI. *See* Adequate intake (AI)

Alli/Xenical (orlistat), for
    weight loss, 57

Allicin. *See* Garlic

Aloe vera, 77

Alzheimer's disease, 53, 62, 72.
    See also Dementia

American ginseng, 95

Amino acids. *See individual*
    amino acids, e.g., Arginine

Anti-aging therapy, 90

Antioxidants, 17

Anxiety, ginseng for, 64

Arginine, 50, 66, 77

Ascorbic acid. *See* Vitamin C
    (ascorbic acid)

Ashwagandha, 62

Astragalus, 50, 77

Athletes, supplement
    consideration in and, 7

Attention-deficit hyperactivity/
    disorder (ADHD)

    nutrients for, 105, 114, 127

    supplements for, 70, 92

B

B vitamins. *See also individual*
    vitamins, e.g., Vitamin B6
    (pyridoxine)

    for brain damage prevention,
      72

    metabolism and, 14

    when to take daily dose, 33

Bacopa monnieri, 72

Berberine. *See* Goldenseal

Beta-carotene, 22, 78–79

Bifidobacterium, 80

Bilberry, 81

Biotin (vitamin B7), 81

Bitter orange, 81

Black cohosh, 82

Blood flow, to brain, 72

Blood pressure levels, managing,
    14, 22, 39, 59, 62

Body mass index (BMI),
    weight-loss drugs and, 37

Bone health, nutrients important
    for, 14, 22

Bovine cartilage, 82

Brain, blood flow to, memory
    and, 72

Brain function, 52

    activities boosting, 73

    supplements boosting, 52,
      68–72

Brain plaques, resveratrol and, 53

Brain volume, preserving, 72

Breastfeeding, nutrient
    deficiency in, 26

Butterbur, 83

C

Cacao, 62

    benefits of, 53, 62

Caffeine, sources of, 36, 39, 70, 99,
    100, 136

Calcium, 84

    for bone health, 14

    deficiency in, 27

    from foods vs. supplements,
      19, 22

    for heart health, 14

Cancer prevention

    nutrients for, 22–23, 35

    supplements for, 52–53

Carotenoids, 78–79

Cat's claw, 85

Celiac disease, nutrient
    deficiency in, 27

Certification, of supplements, 27

Chamomile, 85

Chitosan, 86

    as weight-loss supplement, 56

Chlorogenic acid, 36, 70, 99

Chocolate, benefits of, 53, 62

Choline, 86

Chondroitin, 87

Chromium, 88

CLA. *See* Conjugated linoleic acid
    (CLA)

Cocoa flavanols, 53, 62

Coenzyme Q10, 62–64, 89

Coffee

    for mental alertness, 69, 70

    unroasted beans. *See* Green
      coffee beans

Cognitive alertness. *See* Mental
    alertness

Cognitive decline, age-related, 53

Conjugated linoleic acid (CLA),
    89

    as weight-loss supplement, 56

Contrave (naltrexone/
    bupropion), for weight
    loss, 57

Copper, 89

Cordyceps, 63

Cysteine, 89

D

D-phenylalanine, 115

Dehydroepiandrosterone
    (DHEA), 90

Dementia. *See also* Alzheimer's
    disease

    prevention strategies for,
      68–73

    vitamin deficiencies and, 28,
      35

Depression
    iodine deficiency and, 34
    supplements relieving, 62, 64
    vitamin B12 deficiency and, 28
DHA (docosahexaenoic acid), 72
DHEA (dehydroepiandrosterone),
    90
Diabetes management,
    supplements for, 36, 63–64
Diet, healthy. *See* Healthy diet
Dietary Reference Intakes (DRI),
    16
Docosahexaenoic acid (DHA), 72
DRI (Dietary Reference Intakes),
    16

E
Echinacea, 91
Eicosapentaenoic acid (EPA), 72
Eleuthero (Siberian ginseng), 64
Energy boosters
    exercise, 63
    maca root, 66
    supplements, 62–64
    time spent outdoors, 61
    water, 63
Environment
    natural elements/minerals
        from, 12
    nutrient deficiency and, 32
EPA (eicosapentaenoic acid), 72
Erectile dysfunction,
    supplements for, 66, 112, 136
Essential nutrients, 14
Essential vitamins and minerals,
    6, 12
Estrogen, DHEA and, 100
Estrogen-like substances. *See*
    Phytoestrogens
Evening primrose oil, 91
Exercise
    as energy booster, 63
    for mental alertness, 70
Expert advice, seeking, 42

F
Facial wrinkles, 53

Fat-burning supplements,
    dangers of, 23
Fat-soluble vitamins, 12, 14
Fatigue, supplements reducing,
    60–65
Fenugreek, 66, 92
Fertility, nutrients important
    for, 14
Feverfew, 92
Fish oil, 72, 92
Flavanols, 53, 62
Folate, homocysteine levels and,
    72
Folic acid. *See* Vitamin B9 (folic
    acid)
Food allergy/intolerance/
    sensitivity
    nutrient deficiency and, 27
    supplement consideration in, 7
Foods
    as best source for vitamins,
        18–23
    fortified, 7, 27, 36, 42, 45, 93,
        129
    for healthy diet, 6
    nutrients from, supplements
        vs., 6–7, 12, 18–23
Fortification, 42. *See also* Foods,
    fortified
Free radicals, 17

G
Games
    brain function and, 73
    for mental stimulation, 73
Garlic, 94
Geographic location, nutrient
    deficiency and, 32
Ginger, 94
Ginkgo, 6694
Ginseng
    as energy booster/stress
        reliever, 64, 66
    for mental sharpness, 70
    Panax. *See* Panax ginseng
    for sexual responsiveness, 66
    "Southern." *See* Jiaogulan
Glucomannan, 96

Glucosamine, 97
Glutathione, 97
Gluten malabsorption. *See* Celiac
    disease
Glycine, 98
Goldenseal, 98
Grape seed extract, 98
Green coffee beans, 99
    as weight-loss supplement,
        56, 58
Green tea, 100
    as weight-loss supplement,
        56, 58
Guar gum, 100–101

H
Hawthorn, 102
Healthy diet
    foods for, 6
    multivitamins vs., 40–45
    oversupplementing and, 42, 45
    supplements vs., 6–7, 18–23
Heart health
    nutrients important for, 14
    resveratrol for, 53
Herbal medicine, 72
Herbal supplements, 7
Herbal teas, 85, 136
Herbs, in multivitamins, 27
High-performance mind. *See*
    Mental alertness
Homocysteine levels, managing,
    72, 129
Hoodia, 103
Horse chestnut, 103

I
Immunity
    nutrients important for, 23, 39,
        134, 137
    plant supplements increasing,
        66
Inositol, 104
International unit (IU), 17
Iodine, 104
    deficiency in, 27, 34
    food sources of, 34

Iodized salt, 34
Iron, 105
    deficiency in, 34
    food sources of, 34
Isoflavones, in soy, 122
IU (international unit), 17

J

Jiaogulan, 106

K

Kava, 107
Keto diet, supplement
    consideration in, 7
Kidneys, water-soluble vitamins
    and, 14
Korean red ginseng, 66

L

L-phenylalanine, 115
Labeling, of supplements, 7, 27
Lactobacillus, 107
Lavender, 108
Libido, supplements boosting,
    66–67
Licorice root, 108
Lifestyle/Life stage, supplements
    and, 6–7
Liraglutide (Saxenda), for weight
    loss, 57
Liver, fat-soluble vitamins and, 14
Liver disease, supplements
    causing, 23
Longevity, astragalus for, 50
Low-calorie diets, nutrient
    deficiency in, 27
Lycopene, 22
Lysine, 109

M

Maca root, 66
Macrominerals, 14
Magnesium, 13, 110
    for bone health, 14
    deficiency in, 14, 39

for heart health, 14
Malnutrition, normal aging
    symptoms vs., 48
Manganese, 110
Meat, nutrients in, 12
Medication, for weight loss, 57
Melatonin, 110
Memory
    nutrients/supplements
        boosting, 23, 70, 72, 98, 120,
        122, 127
    vitamin B12 deficiency and, 28
Mental alertness
    cocoa flavanols for, 53, 62
    goals for, 70
    stimulation enhancing, 73
    supplements boosting, 53,
        68–72
Metabolism
    arginine and, 50
    nutrients and, 14
Micrograms (mcg), 17
Milk thistle, 111
Milligrams (mg), 17
Minerals
    dosage amounts/
        measurements, 16–17
    plant foods and, 12
    types of, 14
Multivitamins, 15
    cancer risk and, 45
    fortified cereal and, 112
    healthy eating vs., 40–45
    herbs in, 27
    when to take, 33
Mystery ingredients, in
    supplements, 27

N

Naltrexone/bupropion
    (Contrave), for weight loss,
    57
Niacin (vitamin B3). *See* Vitamin
    B3 (niacin)
Nutrient deficiency
    common forms, 30–39
    following weight-loss surgery,
    37

prevalence in U.S., 32
    screening tests, 35
    susceptibility in people, 24–29
Nutrients
    essential, 14
    from food, 6, 12
    fortified foods and, 7, 27, 36,
        42, 45, 93, 129
    for general health, 14
    intake guidelines, 7, 16–17.
        See also Adequate intake
        (AI); Recommended
        dietary allowance (RDA)

O

Obesity, vitamin D deficiency
    and, 36
Oligomeric. *See* Grape seed
    extract
Omega-3 fatty acids
    from fish/fish oil, 71, 77, 92
    from foods vs. supplements,
        23, 45
    for memory improvement, 72
Orlistat (Alli/Xenical), for weight
    loss, 57
Ornithine, 113
Osteoporosis, supplements for, 90
Outdoors, as energy booster, 61
Oversupplementing, 42
Oxalic acid, manganese and, 110
Oysters, 67

P

P57. *See* Hoodia
Panax ginseng, 95
    for mental sharpness, 70
    as stress reliever, 64
Pantothenic acid (vitamin B5),
    114
Peppermint, 115
Phentermine/topiramate
    (Qsymia), for weight loss, 57
Phenylalanine, 115
Phosphate salts, 146
Phosphorus, 146
    for bone health, 14

Phytoestrogens
  in black cohosh, 82
  in red clover, 119
  soy and, 122
Picky eaters, nutrient deficiency
  in, 27
Polypodium leucotomos extract
  (PLE), skin health and, 52
Pomegranate, 117
Potassium, 117
  for heart health, 14
Pregnancy
  nutrient deficiency in, 26
  supplement consideration in, 7
Prescription medication
  nutrient deficiency and, 28
  for weight loss, 57
Pyridoxine (vitamin B6). *See*
  Vitamin B6 (pyridoxine)
Pyruvate, 58, 117

Q

Q10. *See* Coenzyme Q10
Qsymia (phentermine/
  topiramate), for weight
  loss, 57
Quercetin, 118

R

Raspberry ketone, 119
Recommended dietary allowance
  (RDA)
  calcium, 22
  copper, 89
  defined, 16
  folic acid, 22–23
  fortification and, 42
  iron, 105
  magnesium, 110
  niacin (vitamin B3), 112
  phosphate salts/phosphorus,
    146
  potassium, 147
  selenium, 121
  vitamin A, 129
  vitamin B2 (riboflavin), 119
  vitamin B6 (pyridoxine), 35

Vitamin B9 (folic acid), 93
vitamin B12, 129
vitamin C, 130
vitamin D, 36, 131
vitamin E, 132
zinc, 137
Red clover, 119
Reproductive health, nutrients
  important for, 14
Resveratrol, 53
Riboflavin (vitamin B2), 119

S

Saccharomyces boulardii, 120
Sage, 120
  for mental alertness, 70
Salt, iodized, 34
SAMe, 120
Saw palmetto, 120
Saxenda (liraglutide), for weight
  loss, 57
Screening tests, for nutrient
  deficiency, 35
Selenium, 121
  for reproductive health, 14
  skin health and, 52–53
Semaglutide (Wegovy), for
  weight loss, 57
Sexual responsiveness, ginseng
  for, 66
Siberian ginseng (eleuthero), 64
Silymarin. *See* Milk thistle
Skin cream ingredients, 53
Skin health, aging and, 52–53
Sleep problems, fatigue and, 62
Social life, for mental
  stimulation, 73
"Southern ginseng." *See*
  Jiaogulan
Soy, 122
St. John's wort, 123
Stress, fatigue and, 62
Stress relief, ginseng for, 64
Sulfur, 123
Sun exposure
  free radicals and, 17
  mental sharpness and, 61

skin damage through,
  preventing/reversing,
  52–53, 77, 117
vitamin D and, 27, 32, 35, 36,
  51, 131
Supplements
  anti-aging, 48–53
  availability, 6
  body need considerations, 7
  boosting libido, 66–67
  boosting mental sharpness,
    68–73
  dangers of, 23, 52
  herbal, 7
  labeling of, 7, 27
  oversupplementing, 42
  power of, 46–73
  regulation of, 7
  seeking expert advice on, 42
  shopping for, tips on, 27
  single vs. combination
    products, 7
  for weight loss, 54–59
  well-rounded nutrition vs.,
    6–7, 18–23
Symptoms
  iodine deficiency, 34
  iron deficiency, 34
  magnesium deficiency, 39
  of normal aging, malnutrition
    vs., 48
  vitamin B6 deficiency, 35
  vitamin D deficiency, 35–36

T

Table salt, iodized, 34
Taurine, 124
Tea. *See* Green tea
Testosterone levels, 67
  DHEA and, 100
Thiamine (vitamin B1), 125
Thinking skills, improving, 72–
  73. *See also* Mental alertness
Trace minerals, 14
Tryptophan, 125
Turmeric, 126
Tyrosine, for mental alertness,
  70, 72, 127

U

Ubiquinol, 63
Ubiquinone, 63
Ultraviolet (UV) rays
    PLE and, 52
    vitamin C and, 52
Umckaloabo, 128
Upper Intake Level (UL), defined,
    17

V

Valerian, 128
Vegan diet
    choline source in, 86
    nutrient deficiency in, 26–27
    supplement consideration in, 7
Vegetarian diet
    choline source in, 86
    nutrient deficiency in, 26–27
    supplement consideration in, 7
    vitamin A source in, 22
Vitamin A, 129
    food fortified with, 129
    food source for, 21
    from foods vs. supplements, 22
    for heart health, 14
Vitamin B1 (thiamine), 125
Vitamin B2 (riboflavin), 119
Vitamin B3 (niacin), 112
    for heart health, 14
Vitamin B5 (pantothenic acid),
    114
Vitamin B6 (pyridoxine), 117
    deficiency in, 35
    food sources for, 35

homocysteine levels and, 72
Vitamin B7 (biotin), 81
Vitamin B9 (folic acid), 93
    for female fertility, 14
    food source for, 21
    foods fortified with, 45, 93
    from foods vs. supplements,
        22–23
Vitamin B12, 129
    deficiency in, 28
    homocysteine levels and, 72
    for reproductive health, 14
Vitamin C (ascorbic acid), 130
    essential actions of, 31
    for heart health, 14
    as pollution blocker, 53
    for reproductive health, 14
Vitamin D, 13, 131
    for bone health, 14
    deficiency in, 35–36
    food sources for, 35
    foods fortified with, 27, 36
    screening test for, 35
Vitamin E, 132
    from foods vs. supplements, 23
    for heart health, 14
    for reproductive health, 14
Vitamin K1/Vitamin K2, 133
    for bone health, 14
Vitamins
    dose measurements, 16–17
    essential, 12
    food vs. supplements as source
        for, 18–23
    prenatal, 26
    types of, 12, 14

W

Water, as energy booster, 63
Water-soluble vitamins, 14
Wegovy (semaglutide), for weight
    loss, 57
Weight loss, benefits of, 59
Weight-loss supplements, 54–59
    dangers of, 23
Weight-loss surgery, nutrient
    deficiency following, 37
Whey protein, 58, 134
Workout supplements, dangers
    of, 23
World Health Organization
    (WHO), xanthan gum
    intake, 135

X

Xanthan gum, 135

Y

Yeast (*Saccharomyces boulardii*),
    120
Yerba mate, 136
Yohimbe, 66, 136

Z

Zinc, 137
    for male fertility, 14
    testosterone levels and, 67

DISCLAIMER

Information in *Vitamins & Supplements From A to Z* is provided for awareness and education. Health benefits of various vitamins, minerals, supplements, herbs and foods are the opinion of the author, and there may be differing views on many of the subjects covered, including evolving research, opinions and efficacy. This book is meant to inform and is not a substitute for medical advice and treatment by a physician. Please consult a doctor if you have chronic ailments and do not ingest items to which you have sensitivities, are or may be allergic. Readers should consult a licensed health professional who knows their personal medical history on matters relating to their health and well-being, including potential interactions with other medications, supplements or vitamins you are taking.

CREDITS

COVER nadianb/Shutterstock; Peter Dazeley/Getty Images **2-3** Oppenheim Bernhard/Getty Images **4-5** andresr/Getty Images; AerialPerspective Images/Getty Images;Petegar/Getty Images; rypson/Getty Images; ALEAIMAGE; Westend61/Getty Images; ; Thomas Quack / EyeEm/Getty Images; David Malan/ Getty Images; Emilio Ereza / Alamy Stock Photo; Suparat Malipoom / EyeEm/Getty Images **6-7** Jana Leon/ Getty Images **8-9** fotostorm/Getty Images **10-11** Nicholas Eveleigh / Alamy Stock Photo **12-13** ouh_desire/ Getty Images **14-15** Nicholas Eveleigh / Alamy Stock Photo **16-17** twomeows/Getty Images **18-19** AndreyCherkasov/Shutterstock **20-21** Foxys Forest Manufacture/Shutterstock **22-23** Peter Dazeley/ Getty Images **24-25** Lallapie/Shutterstock **26-27** Stefka Pavlova/Getty Images **28-29** David Malan/Getty Images **30-31** twomeows/Getty Images **32-33** Westend61/Getty Images **36-37** AerialPerspective Images **38-39** Patrick Norman/Getty Images **40-41** j.chizhe/Shutterstock **42-43** Anchiy/Getty Images **44-45** Hinterhaus Productions/Getty Images **46-47** shapecharge/Getty Images **48-49** Westend61/Getty Images **50-51** Westend61/Getty Images **52-53** Westend61/Getty Images **54-55** Mike Kemp/Getty Images **56-57** Peter Dazeley/Getty Images **58-59** Chris Ryan; Getty Images; beijingstory/Getty Images; magnez2/ Getty Images; Olga Kriger / Alamy Stock Photo **60-61** Blend Images - Roberto Westbrook/Getty Images **62-63** andresr/Getty Images **64-65** Alexander Raths/Shutterstock **66-67** Jack Andersen/Getty Images **68-69** JGI/Jamie Grill/Getty Images **70-71** Westend61/Getty **72-73** JGI/Jamie Grill/Getty Images **74-75** Stock-Asso/Shutterstock **76-77** Krug Studios/Getty Images; Sabine Scheckel/Getty Images; sittig fahr- becker / EyeEm; Getty Images; Neil Fletcher/Getty Images **78-79** jon11/Getty Images **80-81** Riou/Getty Images; azure1/Shutterstock; MNS Photo / Alamy Stock Photo; Claudia Totir/Getty Images **82-83** Dorling Kindersley/Getty Images; GK Hart/Vikki Hart/Getty Images; Nicholas Rigg/Getty Images **84-85** DONOT6_ STUDIO/Shutterstock; imageBROKER / Alamy Stock Photo; brozova/Getty Images **86-87** Davies and Starr/ Getty Images; Patricia Soon Mei Yung / EyeEm/Getty Images; MarsBars/Getty Images **88-89** Eric Anthony Johnson/Getty Images; Brad Wenner/Getty Images; James Baigrie/Getty Images, Nodty/Shuttertock; Floortje/Getty Images **90-91** Lauren Burke/Getty Images; Quang Ho/Shutterstock; Carol Sharp/Getty Images **92-93** Michelle Lee Photography/Shutterstock; Nadezhda Nesterova/Shutterstock; TS Photography/ Getty Image; Pixel-Shot/Shutterstock **94-95** Esseffe/Getty Images; DebbiSmirnoff/ Getty Images; NNehring/Getty Images; Ramann/Getty Images **96-97** Joseph Rene Briscoe/Getty Images; DPFishCo/Getty Images; Suparat Malipoom / EyeEm/Getty Images **98-99** IMAGEMORE Co, Ltd./Getty Images; Peter Kindersley/Getty Images; Studio Omg / EyeEm/Getty Images; k_kemruji/Shutterstock **100-101** Daniel Sambraus/Getty Images; govindji/Shutterstock; IMAGEMORE Co, Ltd./Getty Images **102-103** GWX/ Shutterstock; Emilio Ereza / Alamy Stock Photo; Alex Potemkin/Getty Images **104-105** Fernando Trabanco Fotografía/Getty Images; Hiroshi Higuchi/Getty Images; Brian Hagiwara/Getty Images **106-107** Manfred Ruckszio/Shutterstock; HeikeRau/Getty Images; Axel Bueckert / EyeEm/Getty Images **108-109** Petegar/ Getty Images; Science Photo Library/Getty Images; Ekspansio/Getty Images **110-111** dlerick/Getty Images; Maciej Toporowicz, NYC/Getty Images; Gross, Petr/Getty Images; Linda Lewis/Getty Images **112-113** Scaramanga Photography/Getty Images; Claudia Totir/Getty Images **114-115** Eugene Mymrin/Getty Images; StockFood/Getty Images; John E. Kelly/Getty Images **116-117** Vesna Jovanovic / EyeEm/Getty Images, Thomas Quack / EyeEm/Getty Images, Getty Images; Yagi Studio/Getty Images, DustyPixel/Getty Images **118-119** Ly Wylde Photography/Getty Images; julichka/Getty Images; Volosina/Alamy; volkankovancisoy/Getty Images **120-121** David Malan/Getty Images; Seksak Kerdkanno / EyeEm/Getty Images; Dorling Kindersley/Getty Images; UniversalImagesGroup / Contributor/Getty Images; Jim Bastardo/Getty Images **122-123** sot/Getty Images; Alfio Scisetti / Alamy Stock Photo; MirageC/Getty images **124-125** JW LTD/Getty Images; LauriPatterson/Getty Images; Xphi Dech Pha Ti / EyeEm/Getty Images **126-127** imageBROKER / Alamy Stock Photo; Westend61/Getty Images **128-129** Manfred Ruckszio / Alamy Stock Photo; AYImages/Getty Images; Africa Studio/Shutterstock; LOVE_LIFE/Getty Images **130-131** twomeows/Getty Images, Johanna Parkin/Getty Images **132-133** Jonathan Kantor/Getty Images; Destinations by DES - Desislava Panteva Photography/Getty Images **134-135** RobsPhoto/Shutterstock; Akvals/Shutterstock **136-137** Sergio Schnitzler / Alamy Stock Photo; bildagentur-online.com/th-foto / Alamy Stock Photo; ALEAIMAGE/Getty Images **BACK COVER** Blend Images - Roberto Westbrook/Getty Images; Chris Ryan/Getty Images; Stock-Asso/Shutterstock

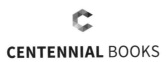

CENTENNIAL BOOKS

An Imprint of
Centennial Media, LLC
1111 Brickell Avenue, 10th Floor
Miami, FL 33131, U.S.A.

CENTENNIAL BOOKS is a trademark of Centennial Media, LLC

All rights reserved. No part of this publication may be reproduced, stored in a retrieval system, or transmitted in any form or by any means (including electronic, mechanical, photocopying, recording, or otherwise) without prior written permission from the publisher.

ISBN 978-1-951274-95-5

Distributed by
Simon & Schuster, Inc.
1230 Avenue of the Americas
New York, NY 10020, U.S.A.

For information about custom editions, special sales and premium and corporate purchases, please contact Centennial Media at contact@centennialmedia.com.

Manufactured in China

© 2021 by Centennial Media, LLC

10 9 8 7 6 5 4 3 2 1

Publishers & Co-Founders Ben Harris, Sebastian Raatz
Editorial Director Annabel Vered
Creative Director Jessica Power
Executive Editor Janet Giovanelli
Features Editor Alyssa Shaffer
Deputy Editors Ron Kelly, Anne Marie O'Connor
Managing Editor Lisa Chambers
Design Director Martin Elfers
Senior Art Director Pino Impastato
Art Directors Olga Jakim, Jaclyn Loney, Natali Suasnavas, Joseph Ulatowski
Copy/Production Patty Carroll, Angela Taormina
Senior Photo Editor Jenny Veiga
Photo Editor Antoinette Campana
Production Manager Paul Rodina
Production Assistant Alyssa Swiderski
Editorial Assistant Tiana Schippa
Sales & Marketing Jeremy Nurnberg